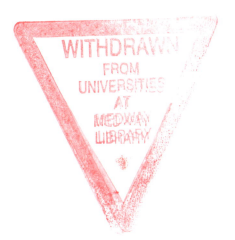

Development and Evaluation of Drugs

From Laboratory through Licensure to Market

Second Edition

Development and Evaluation of Drugs

From Laboratory through Licensure to Market

Second Edition

Chi-Jen Lee, Sc.D.
Center for Biologics Evaluation and Research
U.S. Food and Drug Administration

Lucia H. Lee, M.D.
Center for Biologics Evaluation and Research
U.S. Food and Drug Administration

Cheng-Hsiung Lu, Ph.D.
ChungTai Institute of Health Sciences and Technology
Taiwan

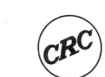

CRC PRESS

Boca Raton   London   New York   Washington, D.C.

Library of Congress Cataloging-in-Publication Data

Lee, Chi-Jen.
    Development and evaluation of drugs : from laboratory through licensure to market / by
Chi-Jen Lee, Lucia H. Lee, Cheng-Hsiung Lu.—2nd ed.
      p. cm.
    Includes bibliographical references and index.
    ISBN 0-8493-1401-1
    1. Drug development. 2. Drugs—Testing, 3. Drugs—Law and legislation—United States.
4. Pharmaceutical industry. I. Lee, Lucia H. II Lü, Zhengziong. III. Title.

RM301.25.L44 2003
615′.19—dc21
                                              2003041011

Visit the CRC Press Web site at www.crcpress.com

© 2003 CRC Press LLC

No claim to original U.S. Government works
International Standard Book Number 0-8493-1401-1
Library of Congress Card Number 2003041011
Printed in the United States of America 1 2 3 4 5 6 7 8 9 0
Printed on acid-free paper

FOREWORD*

Biomedical research has advanced rapidly in the areas of vaccines, traditional plant medicines, recombinant biotechnology, and gene therapy. These scientific advances are anticipated to revolutionize medicine for the prevention and treatment of infections, cancer, and chronic diseases among an increasingly aging society, as well as promote better health and quality of life for all people.

The potential to prevent and treat disease has improved extraordinarily due to the discovery and development of new approaches by academic institutes, government laboratories, and the pharmaceutical industry. The pathogenesis of many disorders has become better understood as our knowledge of immune mechanisms, molecular structures of drugs and biologics, and biotechnology has expanded. Many new classes of vaccines to prevent infections and new therapeutics to treat cancers and chronic diseases have been developed over the past decade.

Disease management has become complicated not only because of the many new drugs, but also because patients with complex diseases are being treated with doses of multiple drugs. Complex therapeutic regimens provide a potential for drug interactions that may induce clinically undesirable adverse reactions. Thus, it is important for health care personnel, biomedical investigators, and pharmaceutical scientists to understand the mechanisms of pharmacokinetic and pharmacodynamic activities and processes of drug evaluation.

The development of new drugs, vaccines, and other biological products requires assurance of the productís efficacy, safety, and purity. It is with this in mind that the authors of *Development and Evaluation of Drugs from Laboratory through Licensure to Market, Second Edition*

---

* The comments of Dr. Walker are his own and do not necessarily reflect an endorsement or opinion of the Food and Drug Administration

have compiled the current procedures and major issues involved in drug development and evaluation. Their text provides both a conceptual approach and specific information about critical steps beginning with drug discovery in the laboratory and progressing to licensure for approval to market. This edition presents the author's examination of how recent advances in pharmaceutical sciences, increased understanding of molecular mechanisms of diseases, and more effective ways to assess drug safety and efficacy have affected the process in which drugs are developed and approved.

This book will constitute a useful reference for investigators in biomedical research, regulatory agencies, the pharmaceutical industry, and health care providers. The approach and specific information available in this volume will prove a most valuable resource.

Richard I. Walker, Ph.D.
Director, Division of Bacterial,
Parasitic, and Allergenic Products
Center for Biologics Evaluation and
Research, FDA

PREFACE

This book has been used as a textbook in the graduate course (Pharmacology 306; Drug Evaluation: From Molecule to Marketplace) at the National Institutes of Health (NIH), Bethesda, MD, to examine the events involved in the evolution of a drug from the chemist's bench to the pharmacist's shelf. It has also been used as an informative reference for scientists in biomedical research, industry, and regulatory agencies. Since the book was first published in 1993, biomedical science, the technological capacity of the pharmaceutical industry, and the drug evaluation process have undergone many advances. These changes necessitate an updated edition.

The revised edition takes a comprehensive look at how recent scientific advances and harmonized regulatory approaches are changing the way in which drugs are discovered, developed, and evaluated.

Greater interest in a rational design of synthetic drugs and developing the "body's own therapeutics," e.g., cytokines as pharmaceutical products, is currently under way. Most of such drugs are protein based, which represents an exciting and growing new family of biologics. Traditional plant medicines are also a topic of heightened public interest. Immunomodulating and antitumor activities observed in polysaccharide fractions of plant medicines support the possibility of plant bioactive molecules as potential therapeutic agents for allergy, cancer, AIDS, and chronic degenerating diseases.

Efforts to streamline differences in market approval procedures for drugs and biologic products internationally are part of the global commitment to deliver new products worldwide. Harmonization of regulatory guidelines is anticipated to facilitate standardization of control tests and simplify the review process for drugs and biological products.

Rational design of new drugs begins with key molecular structures identified and characterized for multiple proteins, polysaccharides, and nucleic acids. Likewise, improvement of existing drugs can translate to increased effectiveness or improved safety profile. The ability to chemically modify cell surfaces and carbohydrate linkages offers exciting prospects for designing the next generation of drugs.

Scientific advances are poised to revolutionize drug discovery. Change is in the air for biomedical research. We hope that this updated edition captures some of the excitement of interdisciplinary pharmaceutical sciences at a time of transition and rapid progress.

The authors thank colleagues and friends, including Dr. Joan C. May, Center for Biologics Evaluation and Research, FDA, and Dr. Mei-Ling Chen, Center for Drug Evaluation and Research, FDA, for their review of the manuscript, comments, and constructive suggestions.

The content of this book is the authors' own and does not represent the official position of their institutions.

Chi-Jen Lee, Sc.D.
Center for Biologics Evaluation and Research, FDA

Lucia H. Lee, M.D.
Center for Biologics Evaluation and Research, FDA

Cheng-Hsiung Lu, Ph.D.
ChungTai Institute of Health Sciences and Technology, Taiwan

THE AUTHORS

Chi-Jen Lee, Sc.D., is Supervisory Research Chemist, Center for Biologics Evaluation and Research, Food and Drug Administration (FDA), Bethesda, MD (1974 to the present, Chief, Polysaccharide and Conjugate Vaccines QC Section).

Dr. Lee graduated in 1957 from National Taiwan University, College of Medicine, School of Pharmacy, with a B.S. in pharmacy. He obtained his Sc.D. in biochemistry in 1966 from Johns Hopkins University, School of Hygiene, Department of Biochemistry. He served as an assistant professor at Rockefeller University, New York City, from 1968 to 1973, and was visiting professor, National Cheng Kung University, College of Medicine, Taiwan, in 1984. He was named honorary professor in 2000 by Inner Mongolia Medical College, China.

Dr. Lee is a member of the American Society for Biochemistry and Molecular Biology, the American Association of Immunologists, and many other professional societies. He has received several FDA Awards of Merit (FDA's highest award, 1986, 1991, and 2001), FDA Commendable Service Awards (1978, 1988), Reward & Recognition Award Certificate and Cash Award (2001), and the Distinguished Achievement Award in Government Service (1988) from National Taiwan University's Alumni Association in North America.

Dr. Lee is the author of *Development and Evaluation of Drugs: From Laboratory through Licensure to Market* (1993, CRC Press) and *Managing Biotechnology in Drug Development* (1996, CRC Press), a co-author of *Polysaccharides in Medicine and Biotechnology* (1996, Marcel Dekker), and the editor of *Professional Frontiers in the 21st Century* (2002, Chinese-American Professionals Association, Greater Washington). Dr. Lee has presented over 40 invited lectures at international and national meetings, universities, and research institutes. He has published more than 150 research papers and abstracts. He served as a thesis director for Ph.D. candidates in the Department of Microbiology, George Washington University Medical Center, Washington, D.C., from 1988 to 1991, and president of the Chinese-American Professionals

Association of Greater Washington from 2001 to 2002. His current major research interests include the immunochemical characterization of bacterial capsular polysaccharides (PSs) and immunostimulating plant PSs, mucosal immunity induced by pneumococcal PS-protein conjugates, and molecular cloning and characterization of the pneumolysin gene.

Lucia H. Lee, M.D., is a medical officer at the Center for Biologics Evaluation and Research, Food and Drug Administration (FDA). Dr. Lee received her medical degree in 1993 from the University of Rochester (New York) School of Medicine. She completed her pediatric training at Johns Hopkins Hospital and then returned to Rochester for a pediatric infectious diseases fellowship. Dr. Lee has published more than 40 research papers and abstracts and her research has been recognized by awards from the Pediatric Infectious Diseases Society and Eli Lilly.

Dr. Lee has extensive training and experience in vaccine and pediatric clinical trial design. She has served in several capacities as a co-investigator and research coordinator for studies conducted in collaboration with the NICHD Pediatric AIDS Clinical Trials Unit and Vaccine Trial Evaluation Unit at the University of Rochester, and continues to be involved in vaccine clinical trial design on both a national and international level. Dr. Lee is also a fellow of the American Academy of Pediatrics and a member of the Pediatric Infectious Disease Society.

Cheng-Hsiung Lu, Ph.D., is Director, Center for Research and Development, ChungTai Institute of Health Sciences and Technology, Taichung, Taiwan. Dr. Lu graduated in 1965 from Taipei Medical College, School of Pharmacy, with a B.S. in pharmacy. He obtained his Ph.D. in microbiology and immunology from George Washington University, Medical Center, Department of Microbiology and Immunology, in 1991. He served as Director, Division of Biologics Quality Control, the National Institute of Preventive Medicine, Taiwan, from 1978 through 1999. From 1999 to 2001, he served as Director, Division of Bacterial Diseases, Center for Disease Control, Taiwan.

Dr. Lu has published more than 40 research papers and abstracts. He has received the Chinese Society of Microbiology Distinguished Scientific paper award in Applied Microbiology in 1998, and several first prize awards in research and development from the Department of Health, Executive Yuan, Taiwan (1998, 1999, and 2000). Dr. Lu is a member of the American Society for Microbiology, the New York Academy of Sciences, and the Chinese Society of Microbiology.

CONTENTS

1

INTRODUCTION

Many drugs in use today have been known for hundreds or thousands of years. These include ephedrine, reserpine, caffeine, opium, etc. The therapeutic properties of these agents were discovered empirically from folklore, traditional medicine, or by screening plants, animals, and microorganisms for pharmacological activity. Ephedrine was used in China for over 5000 years before being introduced into Western medicine in 1924.[1] New drug discoveries, in many cases, are still made empirically by keen observations and alert minds. For example, the discovery of penicillin resulted from the observation of the accidental contamination of a culture of bacterial cells by the mold penicillium.

I. DISCOVERY AND DEVELOPMENT OF DRUGS

A drug is a chemical agent used therapeutically to treat disease. More broadly, a drug may be defined as any chemical agent and/or biological product that affects life processes. Many drugs, including digitalis, cocaine, morphine, and other alkaloids, are of plant origin. Drugs may also be obtained from animal or mineral sources or from microorganisms. Many hormones, such as insulin, growth hormone, and cortico-steroids, for example, are obtained from animal tissues, and various chemotherapeutic antibiotics, e.g., streptomycin, tetracycline, and cephalosporin, are derived from living organisms including bacteria, fungi, and actinomyces. The active ingredients from natural products are isolated and purified by chemical methods.

At the beginning of the 20th century, a metabolic approach was applied to the formulation of new drugs. German bacteriologist Paul Ehrlich contended that since various cells of the body and of various microorganisms could be selectively stained by certain dyes, there must be specific active groups in cells of the human body and in microorganisms to which drugs of the dye type might attach. Such a drug would then act as a "magic bullet," attacking the target cells specifically and killing only the microorganisms while leaving the human body unaffected. Salvarsan, which was developed by Ehrlich on this basis before the antibiotic age, was once the only effective drug for treating syphilis. This approach required a knowledge of the biochemical processes involved in the metabolism of the body. An attempt to cure diseases was then sought by using drugs to alter the body's metabolism. For example, allopurinol was developed for the treatment of gout since it inhibited the enzyme xanthine oxidase that catalyzed the formation of uric acid from xanthine derivatives. Thus, the abnormally high deposition of uric acid in the blood and tissues of gout patients was avoided.

Drug development made a great leap forward with the discovery of antibiotics. In 1928, the Scottish scientist Sir Alexander Fleming found a zone in a culture of bacteria that was caused by the invasion of a mold. Penicillin, the extract from that mold, was shown to cure bacterial infections. The golden age of antimicrobial therapy started in 1941 when the brilliant research of a group of investigators, led by Howard W. Florey and Ernst Chain, purified penicillin and produced quantities sufficient to permit clinical trials. Subsequently, many other antibiotics have been developed. Antibiotics have almost entirely replaced sulfonamides in the treatment of bacterial infection. Because bacteria mutate easily, drug-resistant strains of bacteria develop quickly. As a result, researchers are forced to develop new antibiotics to keep ahead of the steady emergence of drug-resistant strains.

Many modern drugs, however, are synthesized by the techniques of organic chemistry. Even drugs that can be obtained from natural sources, such as the salicylates, are now totally synthesized. Chemical syntheses produce agents of greater purity and at lower cost. The great advantage of synthetic drugs is that changes in the structure of the drug can be made during synthesis, and these changes may enhance the pharmacological activity of the drug or reduce its side effects.[2,3]

As the biochemical and molecular basis of drug actions became better understood, many new drugs have been developed in the past two decades by systematic molecular modification aided by the quantitative structure–activity relationship (QSAR), resulting in the improvement of pharmacokinetic (absorption, distribution, metabolism, and elimination) or pharmacodynamic (mechanism of drug action, cell binding sites) behaviors of drug molecules. All of the effective beta-adrenergic blocking agents are considered to be derivatives of the β-receptor stimulant isoproterenol, which contains an aromatic ring group and a side chain, $ArC–CH(OH)CH_2–NHCH(CH_3)_2$. The side chain with an isopropyl substituted secondary amine determines the interaction with β-receptors, whereas the nature of substituents on the aromatic ring determines whether the effect will be predominantly activation or blockade. Based on studies of the structure–activity relationship, many effective β-adrenergic blockers, such as propranolol, sotalol, etc., were synthesized. Furthermore, many newer antibiotics, e.g., newer generation penicillins and cephalosporins, were developed by systematic molecular modification for the improvement of pharmacokinetic response. Many anticholinergics, H1- and H2-blockers, and analgesic agonists and antagonists were synthesized for the improvement of pharmacodynamic response.

Recently, molecular modeling and computer science are assuming an increasingly important role in understanding the basis of drug-receptor interactions and assisting the medicinal chemist in the design of new therapeutic agents. Computer graphics have emerged as an effective tool for analyzing the three-dimensional structure of macromolecules, and helping in the understanding of molecular interactions.[4] The application of these techniques includes analyses of the interactions of 28 sulfonamide inhibitors of human carbonic anhydrase,[5] mechanism of action and inhibition of thermolysin,[6] and the hormonal activity of steroids.[7] Thus, in the next few years, progress in developing a sound theoretical foundation will make molecular design a realistic aid to the medicinal chemist and protein engineer.

II. SEARCH FOR HEALTH — A DREAM TO CONQUER DISEASES

> Youth is not a time of life — it is a state of mind.
> It is not a matter of red cheeks, red lips and supple knees.
> It is a temper of the will; a quality of the imagination;
> A vigor of the emotions;
> It is a freshness of the deep spring of life.
>
> From *Youth* by Samuel Ullman

Following the rapid progress of medicine and the pharmaceutical sciences, quality of life and well-being have been greatly improved. People strive for youth, health, and happiness. Dreamers imagine a golden age in the remote past, in a far place, free from toil and grief. Optimists put their faith in the future and believe that mankind will overcome illness and control their own destiny through science and technology. However, diseases are still prevalent today.

The hope that health and happiness are within man's grasp flourishes in many cultures. The oldest known medical treatise written in Chinese refers to health as a golden age in the happy past. "In Ancient times," says the Yellow Emperor in the *Classic of Internal Medicine*, "people lived to a hundred years, and yet remained active and did not become weakened in their activities."[8] Ancient philosophers supported the idea that a sound mind in a strong body could be accomplished by following the laws of nature and harmonious life. They believed that the illness was caused by deviating from the natural force and conditions. Thus, the spring of youth and health could be restored by accepting a simple way of life and staying in harmony with nature.

The Taoist philosophy has also profoundly influenced Chinese life and oriental arts by pervading its philosophy with a reverence for nature:

> … Man went to his labors of his own accord in the morning and rested in the evening. People were free and uninhibited and at peace; they did not compete with one another. Contagious diseases did not spread, and long life was followed by natural death.[9]

While modern medicine boasts of so many startling achievements in the health fields, its role appears to be less effective and unique than has been generally claimed. Although the monstrous ghost of infections was inhibited when improved sanitation and drugs were applied to combat microbes, and while many of the terrifying acute diseases, such as typhoid, cholera, and dysentery, have been subdued, many serious microbial diseases have not been eliminated. Encapsulated bacterial diseases, including those caused by meningococci, pneumococci, *Haemophilus influenzae* type b, and others, are still the most prevalent bacterial infections in various areas of the world. The mortality and morbidity of meningitis and pneumonia caused by these organisms are substantially high, despite therapy with antimicrobial agents.[10]

A. Gods of Health and Healing

People usually associate the word *hygiene* with cleanliness. It makes them think of the smell of cresol or phenol solution in the hospital, pasteurized milk, and cookies wrapped with cellophane. The derivation of the word, however, has little relation to cleanliness; rather, hygiene relates to health. The word is derived from Hygeia, a beautiful goddess who once protected and watched over the health of Athens. Hygeia was probably a personification of Greek philosophy, a goddess of reason. Although identified as a goddess of health, she was not involved in the treatment of patients. Rather, she symbolized the protector of health and the concept that humans could remain well if they lived according to reason. To Greeks, Hygeia represented an abstract concept of health, rather than a historical heroine remembered from the great achievements of the past. She did not fight extraordinary battles, like Jeanne d'Arc or Huamulan, a great warrior in Chinese history who substituted herself for her feeble father to fight with the enemy and drove them away. The symbol of Hygeia, like the Statue of Liberty, stands strong in the hearts of the people.[11]

Asclepius, another god involved in healing, was the first physician in Greek mythology. Asclepius achieved his reputation by mastering the skills of surgery and the healing functions of medicinal herbs. His work even became well known beyond Greece. Asclepius appeared as a strong, attractive, and confident young god, accompanied by two lovely maidens, Hygeia on his right, and Panakeia on his left. In contrast to Hygeia, Panakeia became a mighty healing goddess through her knowledge of medicinal herbs and minerals. Her followers are still active today as they search for a *panacea*.

The legends of Hygeia and Asclepius symbolize the never-ending oscillation between two different points of view in medicine – prevention and treatment. For the admirers of Hygeia, health is the reason of natural laws; the most important function of medicine is to discover and teach the natural laws that ensure to people a healthy mind in a healthy body. By maintaining a reasonable life, disease could be prevented. In contrast, followers of Asclepius believe that the main role of a physician is to treat the disease and to restore health by surgical operations to correct any abnormality of the body.

These two complementary concepts of medicine have existed in various cultures and civilizations. The Yellow Emperor's *Classic of Internal Medicine* states that "the ancients followed Tao and the laws of the seasons under the guidance of their sages who were credited with the realization of the value of education in the prevention of disease." Hence even the oldest Chinese medicine emphasizes the importance of complying with natural rules and reasonable behavior for the maintenance of health.

In most primitive societies, disease is considered an invasion by wicked spirits, capricious forces, or misfortune. Ancient Jewish tribes believed that obedience to Jehovah's laws was essential to obtain good health and that any violation of the laws was likely to be punished by disease. Moreover, Jehovah was the supreme healer. In contrast, Hippocratic teachings asserted that both health and disease are under the control of natural laws and reflect the influence exerted by the environment and the way of life. Therefore, health depends on a balance among various internal factors that command the functions of the body and mind; this equilibrium is maintained only when a person lives in harmony with the environment.

Hippocrates (460–377 BCE) has been accepted as the father of medicine; his writings occupy a place in medicine corresponding to that of Shakespeare's dramas and sonnets in the literature of Western society. Hippocrates stands for rational concepts based on the objective knowledge of science; he liberated medicine from the mysterious influences of superstitions and demonic spirits. Hippocratic writings have stressed the relation between environments and the prevalence of various diseases. These writings provided objective descriptions of symptoms, subtle methods of diagnosis, and teachings for dealing with the patient as a person and with his family. For many centuries, Hippocrates has provided the Western world with rational concepts of the philosopher, the objective attitude of the scientist, the practical healing approach of Asclepius, and the sensible idea of prevention symbolized by Hygeia.[11]

In the Hippocratic view, adapting to the environment is essential for health; diseases usually occur when changes in external conditions are too rapid and too violent to allow the adaptive mechanisms of the body to respond. Time and again, Hippocrates emphasized the dangers caused by sudden changes of environment. Furthermore, he taught that anyone well adapted to his environment was not likely to become ill, unless some accident or epidemic occurred. Hippocrates believed that the natural healing forces inside the body could restore the disturbed homeostasis and, therefore, rebuild health. Thus, the crucial role of a physician was to provide an environment and a way of life compatible with the patient's physiological conditions and to supply nutritional foods and proper medicines in order to activate this natural tendency to healing. Indeed, Hippocrates' logical therapeutic policies accomplished for him a great reputation as a physician. His reputation continues in the words carved on his tombstone:

> Here lies Hippocrates, who won innumerable victories over disease with the weapons of Hygeia.

B. The Magic Bullets of Drugs

During the 19th century, the germ theory, generally known as the doctrine of specific etiology of disease, broke the charm of the Hippocratic tradition. The essential part of this theory was that each disease had a well-defined specific cause, and its treatment could effectively be achieved by attacking the causative agent. Many specific microbial agents of disease were discovered one after another by Louis Pasteur, Robert Koch, Von Behring, and other investigators. Thus, many people kindled the hope that all prevalent infections could eventually be controlled by the use of therapeutic sera prepared from specific pathogenic agents. Drugs targeted against these pathogenic agents soon occupied center stage in the minds of medical scientists and investigators, and became the top priority of manufacturers. Whatever the etiology of the disease, these magic bullets of medicine seemed capable of attacking and destroying many of the responsible agents. The dream of conquering a disease is almost always fueled by the discovery and use of an appropriate drug. Such fervent interest and enthusiasm make it possible for active research on chemotherapy to continually leap forward.

Confidence in the magic power of drugs reveals that people can believe in mysterious forces more easily than trusting in reason and rational processes. Although faith in the healing power of ancient gods has weakened, faith in miraculous cures of disease still exists. People want miracles as much today as in the past; they are eager to see the healing power of a spectacular new miracle drug.

The discoveries that led to the wide use of antimicrobial drugs during the last several decades have surpassed ancient medicine both in theoretical and practical importance. However, these accomplishments may not mark the beginning of a new era, but might merely be small advances along the road that medicine has traveled for many years. The sulfonamides, which were considered miracle drugs in the 1930s, are almost totally forgotten by physicians today. The appearance of the new antibacterial drugs cured some acute infectious diseases, e.g., bacillary dysentery, cholera, and gonorrhea. Indeed, the practice of modern chemotherapy has changed the pattern of disease distribution and decreased the mortality rate, but there is no reason to believe that it has completely conquered microbial diseases. Antibiotics, miracle drugs for acute infections after World War II, showed limited efficacy in chronic illness, cancer, and diseases caused by the stresses of life and a malicious environment. Various factors and social environments that induce disease also need to be considered. Further, there are technical limitations in drug development and therapy. Gonorrhea in humans has readily responded to drug therapy since 1935; its etiological agent, the gonococcus, is so vulnerable to penicillin and other chemotherapy that the occurrence of disease can be inhibited in a short time and at a very low cost. Yet, gonorrhea has been prevalent in almost every area and social group in the world. This is because its control involves many physiological, epidemiological, and social factors, and is not solely dependent on effective chemotherapy. These factors include various conditions that allow the continued existence of gonococcus as a carrier or resistant strain in patients, and socioeconomic aspects of the environment that grant loose moral conduct, promiscuity, and juvenile delinquency. These facts imply that drugs cannot be effective in the long run until problems related to pathological and socioeconomic conditions responsible for the disease have been corrected.

Chinese philosopher Lao-Tzu and his Taoist followers advocated that health, joy, and happiness were possible only in a world of primitive simplicity. By merging themselves with their environment and living in harmony with the laws of the four seasons, people could achieve unity with nature in environments such as a peaceful mountain forest, a remote fishing community, or villages and landscapes surrounded by mist-covered pine trees. This life style was not designed to solve the difficulties arising from social conflict and competition. Rather, it attempted to minimize the outgrowth of new problems caused by the stress of life, distress, and insecurity. Concepts in Taoism are rarely achievable in real life; these concepts, however, comprise forever the ideal of human dreams. Health and disease cannot be defined only in terms of anatomical, physiological, or psychological characteristics. Their real estimation appears to be the ability of the individual to function in a manner acceptable to himself or herself as well as to the larger community. The height and body weight of children have been used as general criteria for measuring their state of health, but is size such a desirable measurement? Larger size is not a decisive determinant that a child will live longer, have a greater adaptability to a complex environment, or achieve better opportunities for intellectual growth and success.

People naturally search for health, youth, and happiness. The health that humans require most is not merely a state in which they experience physical strength and psychological maturity. It is, instead, the optimum condition suitable to achieve individual goals in life and social well-being.[11]

III. DRUG DEVELOPMENT IN THE BIOTECHNOLOGY ERA

In the pharmaceutical history of drug development, the period from the 1980s to the 21st century will be referred to as the biotechnology era. Since 1980, numerous proteins that coordinate vital functions of human life and health have been synthesized. Biotechnology produces diverse new products for the pharmaceutical industry and enhances the treatment of disease, as well as improving agricultural yields and diagnostic reagents. The changes wrought by biotechnology involve recombinant DNA (rDNA) technology, genetic engineering, molecular biology, and immunology. For example, the first recombinant human insulin was manufactured by producing the alpha and beta chains separately in *Escherichia coli* and subsequently combining them. The enzymatic conversion of the biosynthetic pro-insulin allows it to be cloned and expressed in yeast. Further, the launch of the thrombolytic agent, tissue plasminogen activator (TPA), has been produced by similar methods. TPA has been used effectively in life-threatening heart disease. In our daily lives, various breeds of poultry and cattle with improved quality have been developed. Furthermore, larger and sweeter oranges, seedless watermelons, as well as hybridizations of colorful flowers and fruits such as the tangelo, a cross between a tangerine and a grapefruit, have come to market.

Biotechnology and related products are likely to have a major impact on many aspects of our lives now and in the future. Among the recent scientific developments are the hepatitis B vaccine and protein drugs that coordinate chemical messages or secreted factors, e.g., interleukin-2 (IL-2); IL-2 is thus a mediator through which immune cells can communicate with each other. There were seven new biological products developed and licensed in FY 2001 by the FDA for use in therapy (Table 1). More than 125 biotechnology products are in various stages of development and clinical trial.[12] These biological products include vaccines, anticoagulants, colony-stimulating factors, erythropoietins, human growth hormones, interferons, interleukins, monoclonal antibodies, tumor necrosis factors, and other products. All of these biological products have been made possible through the biotechnology techniques that allow the isolation, identification, and production of very small amounts of proteins present in the body. Even better, the genes that control protein biosynthesis can be analyzed and their DNA structures sequenced. The isolated gene DNA can be inserted into a bacterial plasmid and cloned into *E. coli* or yeast. This method permits the isolation of specific proteins and their mass production by rapidly growing microorganisms.

Table 1 U.S. FDA-Licensed Biologics in FY 2001

Product (Trade Name)	Manufacturer	Therapeutic Areas
PEG-Intron Peginterferon alfa-2b	Schering Corporation Kenilworth, NJ (1/19/01)	Treatment of chronic hepatitis C in patients not treated with interferon alfa
CroFab Crotalidae Polyvalent Immune Fab (Ovine)	Protherics, Inc. Nashville, TN (12/8/00)	Treatment for venomous snake bites
Myobloc Botulinum Toxin Type B	Elan Pharmaceuticals San Francisco, CA (12/8/00)	Treatment of cervical dystonia to reduce abnormal head position and neck pain
Tripedia Diphtheria & Tetanus & Acellular Pertussis Vaccine Adsorbed	Aventis Pasteur Inc. Swiftwater, PA (3/7/01)	A new formulation of DTaP vaccine
Campath Alemtuzumab	Millennium and ILEX Cambridge, MA (5/7/01)	Treatment of patients with B-cell chronic lymphocyte leukemia
Twinrix Inactivated (Recombinant) Vaccine	SmithKline Beecham Rixensart, Belgium (5/11/01)	Active immunization against hepatitis A and hepatitis B virus
Aranesp Darbepeotin alfa	Amgen, Inc. Thousand Oaks, CA (9/17/01)	Treatment of anemia associated with chronic renal failure

As with various competing technologies, the factor most likely to determine the commercial success of a given technology is its overall cost. The uncertainty of market and investment, and complicated regulatory barriers at an international level, such as rules that favor domestic companies and technology, are key risk factors for biotechnology. In the early period of biotechnology development, newly formed companies were usually managed by scientific investigators. Their lack of management and licensing experience frequently led them to transfer technology to the pharmaceutical industry in exchange for research funding and a 4 to 10% royalty fee on product sales.[13] With growing experience, the larger and better-funded biotechnology companies have arranged and progressed to joint cooperative research and product development. Agreements on strategic alliances have been reached between U.S. and Japanese companies. Examples are those between

Kirin Brewery and Amgen on erythropoietin (EPO) and between Suntory and Schering-Plough on alpha 2-interferon (IFN). These alliances reflect the difficulty of setting up marketing operations in Japan but also indicate the high level of strategic investment in biotechnology by Japanese industry. Commercial prospects for biotechnology products may be viewed and grouped into the following categories:

■ Extraordinary products that are likely to achieve worldwide annual sales in excess of $400 million. In reality, a product that achieves more than $300 million in annual sales is considered extremely successful. For example, Genentech's TPA (Activase) and erythropoietin produced by Amgen and Johnson belong to this category.
■ Major products that may reach annual sales of $200 to 400 million. Biotechnology products in this category include Genentech's human growth hormone, Eli Lilly's human insulin, and many of the colony stimulating factors.
■ Certain products that may reach annual sales of $50 to 200 million, e.g., wound-healing growth factors and streptokinase products.
■ Marginal products that achieve annual sales of less than $50 million, e.g., alpha interferon.

An important parameter in selecting rDNA technology or chemical synthesis is the size of the polypeptide. In general, for the preparation of a peptide below 20 amino acids, chemical synthesis is used. For a peptide between 20 and 50 amino acids, rDNA technology should be considered; above 50 residues an appropriate rDNA route is applied. Calcitonin, for example, has fewer than 50 amino acids and can be prepared by either method, but it appears as if it will be more economical to produce by rDNA technology.

The traditional pharmaceutical approach for the development of drugs entails the screening of large numbers of trial compounds, leading to progressively narrower selection regimes. At this stage, drugs are assumed to be either chemically synthesized organic molecules or natural products. The success of a new drug, after going through all these steps, is based largely on empirical experience or the luck of trial and error. Such an approach, however, is extremely inefficient and expensive. The rational approach to biotechnology drug development utilizes precise knowledge of the key macromolecular reactions to define the structure–activity relationship or receptor–ligand interaction and then to intervene precisely at these reactions. It is the access to these experimental models that enables the rational drug design programs to be effective as well as cost efficient.

Another practical aspect of potential therapeutic proteins is the question of a drug delivery system. The major routes of polypeptide administration are parenteral injections, because after oral administration, polypeptides are rapidly degraded by proteases and aminopeptidases in the gastrointestinal tract. If the therapy is effective for hospital-based or life-threatening situations, delivery by injection will not cause a problem for patients. However, in most other cases, a more suitable administration route is necessary. Although intravenous drug delivery is important clinically, drugs prescribed for oral ingestion are more widely used in the pharmaceutical marketplace. Various attempts have been made to find a more acceptable delivery system than injection, such as the delivery of calcitonin or interferon using a nasal spray. Likewise, a systemic absorption of insulin or glucagon was effectively carried out through the eyes.[14] Thus, new drugs developed by sophisticated biotechnology may require innovative drug delivery systems that are different from the traditional delivery systems in use today.

A. Expanding and Improving Research to Meet Global Health Needs

In the last quarter century, many advances in drug discovery and development have been facilitated by the modern biotechnology synthesis of numerous proteins that coordinate vital functions of human life and health and result from breakthroughs in genomic and proteomic disciplines. Biotechnology research provides methods to identify new moieties for the pharmaceutical industry, enables development of lifesaving medical treatment regimens, and improves agricultural yields and the specificity of diagnostic reagents. Continued application of technologic innovations in biological, pharmaceutical, medical, and agricultural fields offers exciting prospects in all areas of drug development. The outcome of this work-in-progress will most certainly play a major role in shaping the future of pharmaceutical sciences.

Molecular biology concepts applied to established disciplines of medicinal chemistry and pharmaceutical sciences enabled the introduction of more than 50 new therapeutic products into the international marketplace from 1982 to 1996. The products represented 27 unique molecules developed as biological response modifiers, colony stimulating factors, enzymes, hormones, monoclonal antibodies, and vaccines. During 1995 and 1996, more than 1300 biotechnology companies in the U.S. were involved in basic research and product development, and overall, more than 250 molecules were evaluated in human clinical trials.[15]

Adaptations of biotechnology are also apparent in other areas. During the 1980s, the use of transgenic techniques in cell and tissue cultures helped researchers to understand the mechanism of proteins essential for eliciting specific physiological and biochemical responses. For example, erythropoietin is produced by kidney cells, secreted into the blood, and stimulates bone marrow to produce red blood cells. Genome mapping and proteomic sequencing applied to small molecules provide an effective screening method to identify promising drug candidates. Combinatorial chemistry, a powerful tool developed in the 1990s, utilizes a mix-and-match process in which a simple subunit is joined to one or more other subunits in every possible combination.[16] Combinatorial chemistry, which generates compounds via rapid simultaneous, parallel, or automated synthesis, is largely replacing complicated chemical synthesis, a process in which investigators make one compound at a time. Speed — which is reflected in time, money, and an ability to compete — is a key factor in drug development. Combinatorial chemistry is expected to increase the speed of drug discovery and the pace of drug development. It utilizes an automated synthesizing system to form large collections of diverse molecules that can be quickly screened for pharmacological activities and, subsequently, an active compound can be identified for a specific therapeutic target. Thousands of drugs and biologics can thus be generated, screened, and evaluated for further development in a short time.

Completion of the Human Genome Project contributed a comprehensive resource for identification and localization of gene sequence databases and the prospect of continued genome-sequencing research. Extrapolation from detailed genetic maps of 23 human chromosomes, which include the location and identity of individual genes, creates limitless possibilities to detect, treat, and prevent inherited diseases. Characterization of known diseases, and as yet unknown diseases, with a genetic component allows opportunities for early medical intervention. Progress in areas of genetic research and antisense technology are also anticipated. Gene therapy involves the integration of specific genes into the genome of body cells and could ideally be curative for individuals with genetic disorders. Antisense technology incorporates synthetic oligonucleotide sequences with specific mRNA species to inhibit complementary base pairing. Hybridization of the mRNA:antisense strands blocks translation of the mRNA, which effectively provides a method to selectively inhibit gene action.

Improvements in molecular biomedical science techniques have and will continue to significantly impact drug development. A greater understanding of the relationships between protein structure, function, and mechanisms of action is now being realized. Polymerase chain reaction (PCR), transgenic animals and knockout mice, peptide chemistry, recombinant DNA technology, catalytic antibodies, and biosensors are tools that expand the capacity to produce purified drug and biologic products.[17] These bioengineered drugs can be prepared by direct chemical synthesis and, therefore, can be prepared with greater accuracy, at a lower cost, and as a heat-stable formulation. Low-molecular-mass drugs capable of highly specific target interaction can mimic important biological functions and offer possible diagnostic and therapeutic application. Small molecules designed to bind to particular hormone receptors are an attractive option to conventional cancer therapeutic agents. The role of receptor inhibitors in the prevention of pathological processes leading to malignant tumor development is likewise promising. In recent years, there has been an increased interest in developing biologically derived agents as commercially produced pharmaceuticals. Most of such drugs are comprised of proteins and glycoproteins. The number of these biologic products with potential therapeutic application continues to grow.

Modern drug development is a risky, expensive, and lengthy process. At present, the time from discovery of a drug to market availability for a product is estimated to be 8 to 20 years. Start-up research costs in 1994 were estimated to be approximately $7.7 billion for technology companies, and $14.9 billion for traditional drug manufacturers.[16] The overall cost to bring a small-molecule, chemical drug to market is about $350 million. Approximately 5% of available drug candidates considered for evaluation in human studies are successfully approved for commercial use.[18] Development, clinical evaluation, and market approval of biotechnology products is a similar process. The success rate for market approval of a biological product is similar to that for drug candidates. From a regulatory standpoint, the standard time in the U.S. for reviewing all data supporting market approval of a new drug in 1993 and 1994 was 1.7 years, compared to 3 years in Europe and 4.7 years in Japan.[19]

The interest in developing biotech-derived products is reflected in their projected market value. In 1993, the estimated worldwide sales of biopharmaceuticals were approximately $5 billion, of which erythropoietin accounted for $1.2 billion and alpha-interferon accounted for over $0.5 billion. Successful development of one or two "gangbuster" products substantially increases investment interest. In 1997, the growth potential for biopharmaceuticals had increased to more than $7 billion. By 2003, the global biopharmaceutical market is projected to reach approximately $30 to 35 billion and represents approximately 15% of the overall world pharmaceutical market.[17]

During the early 1980s, there was a tremendous influx in capital investment for biotechnology companies. Cooperative partnerships were formed in biotechnology comprised of private, national, and international organizations with a public health interest. Financial support from the National Institutes of Health (NIH), the National Science Foundation (NSF), the Centers for Disease Control (CDC), and the Food and Drug Administration (FDA) encouraged basic research in areas related to biomedicine and biotechnology. International organizations, such as the Japan International Cooperation Agency (JICA), Japan International Development Organization (JIDO), the Organization for Economic Cooperation and Development (OECD), and European Community (EC), also supported research and development in the biopharmaceutical disciplines. In the global biotechnology arena, concerns have been raised that international alliances could place the U.S. at a competitive disadvantage. Available U.S. technology, developed with support from the U.S. government, could easily be obtained and rapidly distributed to companies in Japan and Europe. Accelerated imports of agricultural, medical, and pharmaceutical products from these resources might oversaturate the U.S. domestic market.[20]

Financial support greatly diminished after the stock market crash in October 1987. Due to economic uncertainty, primary sources of funding for biotechnology firms shifted from individual investors to pharmaceutical manufacturers and large corporations. Since biotechnological capability was still relatively new to the pharmaceutical research repertoire, large pharmaceutical companies were at a disadvantage compared with established biotechnology firms to skillfully develop novel products. In the process of expanding research facilities and training investigators to develop expertise in specific technologies, large companies formed long-term alliances with established biotechnology firms. Despite concerns regarding long-term economic instability, additional alliances between U.S. companies and companies abroad will likely develop. Economic growth in Asia's newly industrialized countries has been remarkably successful. Stability is due in part to solid investment in manufacturing industries and aggressive marketing of exports. Continued achievement by Asian nations in areas of applied biotechnology is the result of strong local government support, utilization of available financial resources, and enthusiastic industry commitment.

B. Genome Structure for Understanding the Encoded Proteins

The Human Genome Project, which has mapped every gene, will affect every branch of molecular biology and drug development. The complete DNA sequencing of humans and animals will decipher many important questions as to how to treat a wide range of diseases and medical disorders through understanding the proteins encoded by the genes. Proteins make up the structural basis of the human body and the various enzymes that carry out the biochemical functions of life. Proteins are composed of amino acid units linked in a long string of peptides folding in a way that determines the protein's activities. The order of amino acid structure is determined by the DNA sequence of the gene, through the intermediate molecule of RNA.

For understanding the basic functions of life, it is important to elucidate all the proteins produced within a human body, grasp how the genes that encode the proteins are expressed, how genes vary within our species and other animal species, and how DNA sequences affect biologic characteristics of proteins. Genomics will promote the understanding of mechanisms involved in preventive, diagnostic, and therapeutic medicine. Investigators will comprehend the molecular basis of diseases, be able to prevent them in many cases, and design individual therapies to treat medical disorders. Once the DNA sequence of the human genome is known, scientists will be able to identify common genetic variations and examine how particular variations correlate with risk for disease as well as the interaction between genes and environmental influences such as diet, infection, and pollution.

In the near future, novel drugs will become available that are derived from a detailed molecular understanding of chronic diseases such as diabetes and high blood pressure. The drugs will target molecules logically and more accurately and thus will reduce side effects. Drugs for treatment of cancer and cardiovascular diseases will routinely be matched to a patient's likely response, as predicted by molecular fingerprinting. Diagnosis of many abnormal conditions will be more thorough and specific. For example, a patient with high cholesterol will know which genes are responsible and what diet and medicines will work best. When people become ill, therapists will examine individual genes to provide precise and customized treatment. The average life span will reach 90 to 95 years, and understanding of human aging genes will expand the maximum length of human life.[21,22]

Drug companies collect the genetic know-how to make medicines tailored to specific genes. This is called *pharmacogenomics*. In years to come, a pharmacist may give a patient cholesterol-reducing and blood pressure medicines based on the individual's unique genetic profile. Blood tests that reveal specific disease–gene mutations forecast the chances of developing abnormal conditions such as Huntington's disease. Furthermore, gene therapy directly introduces healthy genes into a patient's body to restore the morbid functions of hereditary diseases.

In the spring of 2000, all attention was focused on the first finish line in the genome, a draft sequence of the 100,000 genes inside the human body. The Human Genome Project team separated out the 23 pairs of chromosomes that hold human genes. Scientists then cut off pieces of DNA from every chromosome, identified the sequence of DNA bases, and matched each small piece to the DNA on either side of it in the chromosome. They gradually manipulated the sequences for individual gene segments, complete genes, whole chromosomes, and the entire genome.

The genome investigators focused on similarities among humans. They considered that 99.9% of genes match perfectly among all individuals, but the remaining 0.1% of genes vary. It is in these variations, even a simple *single-nucleotide polymorphism* (SNP), that drug companies are most interested. Because of these slight genetic variations, many drugs work only in 30 to 50% of the human population. A drug that treats and saves one person might harm another. The type II diabetes drug, Rezulin, which has been linked to more than 60 deaths worldwide from liver toxicity, is an example. In the future, a simple genetic test might determine whether a patient is likely to be treated effectively or whether the individual faces the risk of serious side effects by the same drug.[23,24]

A multimillion dollar industry has emerged around turning initial genome data into knowledge for developing new drugs. The new discipline of *bioinformatics* has combined computer science and biomedicine for finding better drug targets earlier in the drug discovery process. Pharmaceutical companies make great efforts in collecting and storing data, searching databases, and interpreting the data. The efficiency of finding drug targets could trim the number of potential therapeutics proceeding through a company's clinical trials, thus significantly reducing overall costs.

Once the Human Genome Project officially started in 1990, the volume of DNA-sequence data in GenBank began to grow exponentially. Other public and private databases contain information on gene expression, tiny genetic differences among individuals, the structures of various proteins, and maps of how proteins interact. The important operations in bioinformatics involve searching for similarities, or homologies, between a newly sequenced piece of DNA and previously sequenced DNA segments from various organisms. Identifying near-matches allows scientists to predict the type of protein the new sequence encodes. This procedure leads to finding better drug targets early in drug development and discontinue the studies on the dead end targets.

Bioinformatics has been utilized in research on cathepsin K, an enzyme that might turn out to be an important target for treating osteoporosis, a disease caused by the breakdown of bone. In 1993, SmithKline Beecham (SKB) asked scientists at Human Genome Sciences to help analyze some genetic material isolated from the osteoclast cells of people with bone tumors. The scientists sequenced the sample and conducted database homology searches to look for matches that would give them a clue to the proteins that the sample's gene sequences encoded. Later, they discovered that a particular sequence was overexpressed by the osteoclast cells and that it matched those of a previously identified class of molecules, cathepsins.

The application of bioinformatics produced, in just weeks, a promising drug target for the company that other laboratories could not have found in years. GKB (formerly SKB) is now trying to find a potential drug that blocks the cathepsin K target. Searching for compounds that bind to and induce the desired effect on drug targets still takes place in the biochemical laboratory, whereas evaluations of biological activities, toxicity, and absorption can take years. But now, the new bioinformatics tools utilize enormous amounts of data on protein structures and bio-molecular pathways in early aspects of drug development.

In bioinformatics, pharmaceutical companies experience the beginning of the scientific revolution. The revolution involves many different players with different approaches. Some bioinformatics companies, e.g., Lion Bioscience in Germany, provide their products and services to many users in genomics, biotechnology, and pharmaceutical companies by creating custom software and offering consulting services. Other firms target small or academic users. Web businesses such as Double Twist and eBioinformatics in California offer one-stop Internet shopping. Large pharmaceutical companies have also sought to enforce in-house bioinformatics investments. Many have established entire departments to integrate and service computer software and facilitate database access across various departments including new product development, formulation, toxicology, and clinical trials. To integrate bioinformatics throughout their companies, "big pharms" also forge strategic alliances, enter into licensing agreements, and acquire smaller biotechnology companies.[25,26]

With all the DNA that codes for a human deciphered, the challenge then becomes when and where these genes are activated and what are the properties of the proteins the genes encode. Although every cell in the body contains all of the DNA code for maintaining biochemical functions, many of these genes are never activated or transcribed into mRNA. Various other genes are turned on or off at different times, according to the tissue they are in and their role in the body. The DNA sequence of the human genome therefore explains only a small fraction of the mechanism about what a specific cell is doing. Instead, scientists must also examine the processes on production of mRNA (*transcriptome*) and proteins (*proteome*).

One of the technologies for studying human transcriptome is based on nail-size glass chips called microarrays that are coated with a thin layer of cDNAs (which represent complementary DNAs artificially translated back by mRNAs but without the noncoding sequence gaps, or introns, found in the original genomic DNA). To use the system, mRNA is isolated from the cellular sample, tagged with a chemical marker, and coated over the chip. By observing where the sample mRNA matches and binds to the cDNA on the chip, scientists can identify the mRNA sequences in the sample. Using these chips, human cell samples can be analyzed to identify more than 60,000 different human mRNA or screen cells for approximately 1700 human mRNA related to cancer. The National Cancer Institute has identified more than 50,000 genes that are active in one or more cancers; 5692 genes are active in breast cancer cells, including 277 that are not active in other tissues. Compounds reacting with molecules contained in the proteins produced by these 277 genes might serve as effective anticancer drugs with fewer side effects than current chemotherapeutic agents.

Furthermore, the proteins are more useful and effective drug targets. Within the next decade pharmaceutical companies will deal with evaluating up to 10,000 human proteins against which new drugs might be developed. Scientists in DNA-sequencing research are interested in the study of protein expression or *proteomics*. Investigators at Myriad Genetics (Salt Lake City, UT) analyzed BRCA genes that contribute to breast and ovarian cancer. Later, Myriad made an agreement with Roche worth up to $13 million to lend its proteomics techniques to finding targets for potential cardiovascular disease drugs.

Protein chips have been used for studying the expression of proteins. One of the initial applications of Ciphergen's (Fremont, CA) protein chips is in finding early markers for prostate cancer. By using Ciphergen's system, investigators have identified 12 candidate markers for benign prostate disease and six markers for prostate cancer. Tests based on the proteomics technique might be better at discriminating between benign and cancerous prostate conditions than the currently used prostate specific antigen (PSA) determination.[27,28]

REFERENCES

1. Chen, K.K. and Schmidt, C.F., Ephedrine and related substances, *Medicine* (Baltimore), 9, 1, 1930.
2. Burgen, A.S.V., The road to rational drug design, in *Innovative Approaches in Drug Research*, Harms, A.F. (Ed.), Elsevier Publishing Company, 1986, 1.
3. Sarel, S., Mechoulam, R., and Agranat, I. (Eds.), Rational drug design, in *Trends in Medicinal Chemistry '90*, Blackwell Scientific, Oxford, 1992, 55.
4. Marshall, G.R., Computer-aided drug design, *Annu. Rev. Pharmacol. Toxicol.*, 27, 193, 1987.
5. Vedani, A. and Meyer, E.F. Jr., Structure-activity relationships of sulfonamide drugs and human carbonic anhydrase C: modeling of inhibitor molecules into the receptor site of the enzyme with an interactive computer graphics display, *J. Pharm. Sci.*, 73, 352, 1984.
6. Smith, G.H., Hangauer, D.G., Andose, J.D., Bush, B.L., Fluder, E.M., et al., Intermolecular modeling methods in drug design: modeling the mechanism of peptide cleavage by thermolysin, *Drug Inf. J.*, 18, 167, 1984.
7. Hendry, L.B., Bransome, E.D. Jr., Lehner, A.F., Muldoon, T.G., Hutson, M.S., and Mahest, V.B., The stereochemical complementarity of DNA and reproductive steroid hormones correlates with biological activity, *J. Steroid Biochem. Mol. Biol.*, 24(4):843, 1986.
8. Ilza, V., Huang Ti Nei Ching Su Wen, *The Yellow Emperor's Classic of Internal Medicine*, Williams & Wilkins, Baltimore, 1949, 253.
9. Needham, J., The Tao chia (Taoists) and Taoism, in *Science and Civilization in China. Vol. 2, History of Scientific Thought*, Cambridge University Press, Cambridge, 1956.
10. Lee, C.J., Bacterial capsular polysaccharides — biochemistry, immunity and vaccine, *Mol. Immunol.*, 24:1005, 1987.
11. Dubos, R. and Dubos, J., Hygeia and Asclepius, in *Mirage of Health*, Harper & Brothers, New York, 1959, 109.
12. Pharmaceutical Manufacturers Association, Biotechnology medicines in development, *Gene. Eng. News*, 27, 1992.
13. Gordon, S.L., Overview of the commercial prospects for biotechnology products in health care, in Copsey, D.N. and Delnatte, S.Y.J. (Eds.), *Genetically Engineered Human Therapeutic Drugs*, Macmillan, New York, 1988, 137.
14. Chiou, G.C.Y., Systemic delivery of polypeptide drugs through ocular route, *Annu. Rev. Pharmacol. Toxicol.*, 31:457, 1991.

15. Pharmaceutical Research and Manufacturers of America, *Biotechnology Medicines in Development,* Washington, D.C., 1996.
16. Lee Jr., K.B., Burrill, G.S., Biotech 96, The Industry Annual Report, 1995, Ernst and Young LLP.
17. Sindelar, R.D., Additional biotechnology-related techniques, in *Pharmaceutical Biotechnology,* Crommelin, D.J.A. and Sindelar, R.D. (Eds.), Harwood Academic Publishers, Amsterdam, 1997, 123–166.
18. Shapiro, B., Merck and Co., The impact of biotechnology on drug discovery, 9th International Congress of Immunology, San Francisco, 1995.
19. Struck, M.M., Biopharmaceutical R & D success rates and development times, *Bio/Technology,* 12, 674–677, 1994.
20. Yuan, R.T. and Dibner, M.D., *Japanese Biotechnology: A Comprehensive Study of Government Policy, R & D, and Industry,* Macmillan, London, 1990.
21. Collins, F.S. and Jegalian, K.G., Deciphering the code of life, *Sci. Am.,* 281(6): 86–91, 1999.
22. Collins, F.S., Genome project, *N. Engl. J. Med.,* 341:28–37, 1999.
23. Green, E., The Human Genome Project and its impact on the study of human disease, in *Metabolic and Molecular Bases of Inherited Disease,* 8th ed., Scriver, C.R. (Ed.), McGraw-Hill, New York, 2000.
24. Pennisi, E., Are sequencers ready to annotate the human genome? *Science,* 287:2183, 2000.
25. Searls, D.B., Using bioinformatics in gene and drug discovery, *Drug Discovery Today,* 5:135–143, 2000.
26. Howard, K., The bioinformatics gold rush, *Sci. Am.,* 283(1):58–63, 2000.
27. Abbott, A., A post-genomic challenge: learning to read patterns of protein synthesis, *Nature,* 402:715–720, 1999.
28. Ezzell, C., Beyond the human genome, *Sci. Am.,* 283(1):64–69, 2000.

2

DRUG EVALUATION FROM LABORATORY THROUGH LICENSURE TO PHARMACIST'S SHELF

Drug development is a complicated, time-consuming, and costly process. At present, a new drug identified in the laboratory generally takes 8 to 20 years to achieve market approval. After product approval, an additional 18 months may be needed before a product becomes available to the public. For any potential drug candidate, success rates for market approval and global demand are unpredictable. Various strategies are applied by the pharmaceutical industry in their efforts to identify new drugs. These approaches range from repeated random screening of chemical agents and biological materials to knowledge-based drug design. When a potential new drug has been discovered, initial testing for biochemical characterization provides preliminary assessments of efficacy and safety for the intended indication.

Traditionally, the drug discovery process has relied on screening large numbers of biological specimens to identify potential candidates. Prior to the 1950s, crude substances were initially extracted from plants. Plant derivatives were eventually modified to active compounds found in digitoxin, ephedrin, and taxol. Large quantities of the plant material were collected, and purified to yield the active principal, known as a "lead compound." Chemists then attempted to modify the lead compound to make it more pharmacologically active, reduce potential toxicity, or change its hydrophobicity so it can easily pass through cell membranes. These properties all render the compound more attractive as a pharmaceutical agent. Drug discovery, in most cases, relates to an efficient, insightful interpretation of biochemical knowledge and logical application to biologic function. Purification of crude substances was gradually replaced by large-scale systematic screening of natural and synthetic compounds. Today, more sophisticated and efficient knowledge-based strategies are utilized to identify new compounds. Structure-based drug design using computer modeling is also used to simulate chemical modifications. In this way, modification of an existing leading drug or designing a new drug is achieved without physically manipulating every compound.

Continuing advancements in molecular biology and biomedicine have facilitated our understanding of the molecular mechanisms involved in health and disease. A clear understanding of biologic mechanisms of action and pathological processes, which maintain health or result in disease, often leads to important approaches and strategies to control that disease. The cause of many chronic diseases, such as cancer and immunodeficiency illness, are frequently multifactorial and involve complex feedback mechanisms. Within the body's own immune repertoire, cytokines, interferons, and interleukins that stimulate positive responses have proven to be effective in treating such complex diseases. An understanding of the biochemical actions or mechanisms of disease does not, however, automatically translate into an effective treatment. Biologic products, such as cytokines, exhibit multiple functions depending on the type of cell population involved. In addition, cytokine production is regulated by complex regulatory feedback mechanisms. Pattern-specific recognition and variable outcome makes it difficult to predict the desired response of this biologic product on overall body function.

In the U.S., the Food and Drug Administration (FDA), a regulatory agency for drugs and biologic products, the National Institutes of Health (NIH), the largest institution for biomedical research, and the Centers for Disease Control and Prevention (CDCP), which conduct epidemiologic surveys of diseases, all belong to the Public Health Service, Department of Health and Human Services (Figure 1A). The FDA (Figure 1B) is subdivided into several centers. The Center for Drug Evaluation and Research (CDER; Figure 1C) evaluates drug safety and efficacy, and is responsible for ensuring accurate product labeling. The Center for Biologics Evaluation and Research (CBER) performs similar duties for biological products intended for human use. Manufacturing information includes specifications and analytic methods for identity,

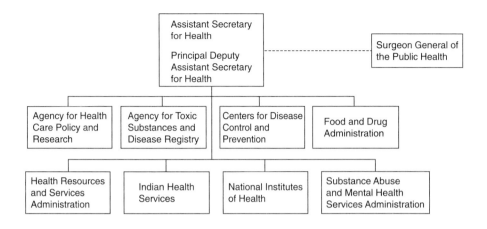

Figure 1A Organization of the Public Health Service, Department of Health and Human Services (From Lee, C.J., *Managing Biotechnology in Drug Development*, CRC Press, Boca Raton, 1996, 18. With permission.)

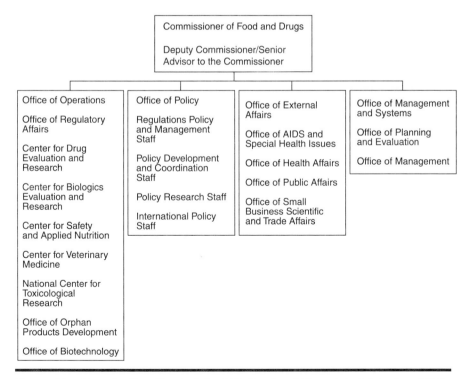

Figure 1B Organization Chart of the U.S. Food and Drug Administration (FDA) (From Lee, C.J., *Managing Biotechnology in Drug Development*, CRC Press, Boca Raton, 1996, 18. With permission.)

Office of the Center Director

Office of Executive Program
- Executive Operations Staff
- Review Standards Staff
- Advisors and Consultants Staff
- Information Management Program

Office of Counter-Terrorism and Pediatric Drug Development
- Division of Pediatric Drug Development
- Division of Counter-Terrorism

Office of Regulatory Policy
- Division of Regulatory Policy I
- Division of Regulatory Policy II
- Division of Information Disclosure Policy

Office of Management
- Division of Management and Budget
- Division of Management Services

Office of Training and Communication
- Division of Training and Development
- Division of Drug Information
- Division of Public Affairs
- Division of Library and Information Services

Office of Compliance
- Division of Labeling and Nonprescription Drug Compliance
- Division of Manufacturing and Product Quality
- Division of Prescription Drug Compliance and Surveillance

Office of Information Technology
- Quality Assurance Staff
- Technology Support Services Staff
- Division of Data Management and Services
- Division of Infrastructure Management and Services
- Division of Appliance Development Services

Office of Medical Policy
- Division of Scientific Investigations
- Division of Drug Marketing

Office of Pharmaco-epidemiology and Statistical Science

  Office of Drug Safety
  - Division of Surveillance, Research, and Comm. Support
  - Division of Medication Errors and Technical Support
  - Division of Drug Risk Evaluation

  Office of Biostatistics
  - Quantitative Methods and Research Staff
  - Division of Biometrics I
  - Division of Biometrics II
  - Division of Biometrics III

--- *continued*

Figure 1C   Organization Chart of the Center for Drug Evaluation and Research, FDA (FDA Location Directory, U.S. Department of Health and Human Services, Public Health Service, FDA, Washington, D.C., 1996.)

Office of New Drugs
  Office of Drug Evaluation I
    - Division of Neuropharmacological Drug Products
    - Division of Oncology Drug Products
    - Division of Cardio-Renal Drug Products
  Office of Drug Evaluation II
    - Division of Pulmonary Drug Products
    - Division of Metabolic and Endocrine Drug Products
    - Division of Anesthetic, Critical Care, and Addiction Drug Products
  Office of Drug Evaluation III
    - Division of Gastrointestinal and Coagulation Drug Products
    - Division of Reproductive and Urologic Drug Products
    - Division of Medical Imaging and Radiopharmaceutical Drug Products
  Office of Drug Evaluation IV
    - Division of Anti-Viral Drug Products
    - Division of Anti-Infective Drug Products
    - Division of Special Pathogen and Immunologic Drug Products
  Office of Drug Evaluation V
    - Division of Anti-Inflammatory, Analgesic, and Ophthalmologic Drug Products
    - Division of Dermatologic and Dental Drug Products
    - Division of Over-the-Counter Drug Products
Office of Pharmaceutical Science
  Office of Clinical Pharmacology and Biopharmaceutics
    - Division of Pharmaceutical Evaluation I
    - Division of Pharmaceutical Evaluation II
    - Division of Pharmaceutical Evaluation III
  Office of Generic Drugs
    - Division of Chemistry I
    - Division of Chemistry II
    - Division of Bioequivalence
    - Division of Labeling and Program Support
  Office of New Drug Chemistry
    - Microbiology Team
    - Division of Drug Chemistry I
    - Division of Drug Chemistry II
    - Division of Drug Chemistry III
  Office of Testing and Research
    - Laboratory of Clinical Pharmacology
    - Division of Applied Pharmacology
    - Division of Product Quality Research

Figure 1C (continued)   Organization Chart of the Center for Drug Evaluation and Research, FDA (FDA Location Directory, U.S. Department of Health and Human Services, Public Health Service, FDA, Washington, D.C., 1996.)

strength, quality, purity, bioavailability, and stability data. Product potency refers to the demonstration of the pharmacological activity or biological effect, by *in vitro* or *in vivo* testing for each lot or batch. Safety of the investigational product is assessed from detailed review of the manufacturing process and test procedures, clinical study results, and control testing the bulk and final lots of product before release to market. Efficacy is examined in one or more controlled clinical trials. Market approval is granted if scientific and clinical data provide sufficient evidence to demonstrate safety and efficacy for the proposed indication. Following licensure, monitoring of product safety and effectiveness continues during post-marketing surveillance of the target population.

The consequences of costly and lengthy drug development are not limited to the pharmaceutical industry. For pharmaceutical companies, decreased and delayed returns on investments translate to less funding for new research and development. For patients with illnesses unresponsive to conventional medical treatment, insurance company concerns about potential liability for unexpected events may limit patient access to promising investigational treatments. For the general consumer, increasing drug costs contribute to the rising cost of health care. For any regulatory agency, redundant clinical studies and conventional methods of evaluating efficacy may no longer be possible. Alternate and more efficient ways to demonstrate efficacy are needed to assess drug safety and efficacy. In addition, regulation of biopharmaceutical products poses additional challenges in review, research, policy development, and compliance activities. As the FDA re-evaluates its requirements for approving conventional drugs and new biopharmaceutical products, re-evaluation of priorities among other interested parties may also occur.

Prior to the 1990s, regulation was based mainly on the premise that traditional biological products, such as viral and bacterial vaccines, blood products, and allergenic extracts, were not uniform mixtures. The precise chemical nature of these products was considered impossible to define. In contrast, for traditional chemical drugs, molecular structures could be clearly defined. Chemical drugs could also be purified, characterized, and identified by accurate and reproducible methods. Thus, a product was categorized as a biologic or chemical drug depending on the manufacturing process. In addition, regulation of biologic products required simultaneous issuance of an establishment license and a product license. The transition to analytical methods, which enabled characterization of complex molecules, resulted in streamlining the evaluation of quality and therapeutic use of biologic products more like traditional chemical drugs.

Progress in biomedicine, particularly in areas of genomics, immunology, rDNA technology, and vaccinology, has enabled development of more biological products. The 1990s represented a decade of dramatic changes in the regulation of biopharmaceuticals in the U.S. since the health-related law was established in 1944. Government initiatives began in 1993 and emphasized performance-based management for agencies involved in review work. Reinventing Government I (REGO I) outlined four basic principles: first, cut obsolete regulations; second, reward results, not red tape; third, get out of Washington and create grass roots partnerships; fourth, negotiate, don't dictate. REGO II initiatives were introduced in 1995. The major regulatory reforms included:

- Elimination of many requirements for FDA pre-approval of manufacturing changes for drugs and biologics
- Institution of a new policy to permit the use of small-scale and pilot manufacturing facilities during development of biological products in support of eventual product approval
- Revision of labeling requirements for biological products to partially harmonize drug and biologics labeling regulations
- Revision of requirements to submit an environmental assessment analysis for all application submissions

Approaches to the use of pilot facilities and reduction of postlicensure reporting requirements were adapted on the basis of improvements in the chemical characterization of drugs and biologics.

REGO IIb further modified regulations pertaining to drugs made from biotechnology. It consisted of the following major reforms:

- Elimination of the requirement for an Establishment License Application (ELA) for therapeutic biotechnology products that are considered to be well characterized
- Elimination of the requirement that Center for Biologics Evaluation and Research (CBER), FDA, release every lot of all wellcharacterized biotechnology product after licensure
- Development of a harmonized application format for well-characterized products and, eventually, for all human drugs and biologics
- Elimination of the requirement to pre-approve promotional labeling for biologics

- A commitment by the FDA to review and respond to submitted IND within 30 days of receipt
- Revision of the requirement to name a single individual, the responsible head, to manage control of a biologics manufacturing establishment in all matters

These initiatives served to harmonize the regulatory requirements for drugs and biologics that are well characterized. REGO IIb proposed the most significant reform effort to define a well-characterized biological product. The definition of a well-characterized product was provided as follows: a chemical entity or entities whose identity, purity, impurities, potency, and quantity can be determined and controlled. For example, the identity of rDNA products is determined by the chemical properties of primary amino acid sequence and secondary structure, e.g., disulfide linkages, as well as post-translational modifications, e.g., glycosylation and phosphorylation. Purity is assessed by identification and quantitative analysis of impurities, if possible. The potency and quantity of the product are evaluated by measuring biological activity and amount of product.

In 1996, the "Elimination of the establishment license application for specified biotechnology and specified synthetic biological products" was published.[1] Regulatory flexibilities were extended to four categories of specified products: (1) therapeutic DNA plasmid products; (2) therapeutic synthetic peptide products of fewer than 40 amino acids; (3) monoclonal antibody products in *in vitro* use; and (4) therapeutic products derived from rDNA.

The revised regulatory policy further integrated the requirements for drugs and biologic products. Several steps were proposed:

- Finalizing the CMC guidance documents for traditional biological products. The Biologics License application will be utilized as a single application for all biologics
- Refining the harmonized application format to be applicable to the submission of all drugs and biologics, regardless of their ability to be characterized
- Harmonizing application review and inspection procedures for drugs and biologics

Several regulatory policies for well-characterized biologics were implemented to meet the commitments initiated by regulation and legislation proposed during the 1990s.

I. DRUG EVALUATION PROCESS AND LICENSURE

A. Drug Discovery and Preclinical Research

Preclinical research, the initial process of drug development, is intended to provide a preliminary assessment of a product's pharmacokinetics, pharmacodynamics, dose–response profiles, and toxicological potential. In addition to providing basic information about the pharmacology and safety of the test drug, preclinical studies determine the optimal formulation and dose for Phase I trials, identify potential toxic adverse effects, and provide the rationale for the proposed therapeutic indication. Figure 2 shows various stages of development and regulation of drugs and biological products.

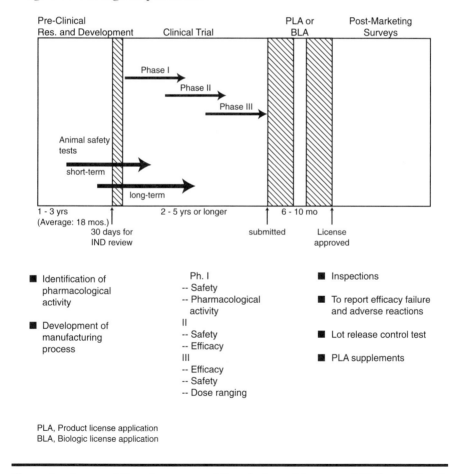

Figure 2   Stages of Development and Regulation of Drugs and Biological Products (From Lee, C.J., *Development and Evaluation of Drugs from Laboratory through Licensure to Market*, CRC Press, Boca Raton, 1993. With permission.)

Approval to initiate human clinical studies is based largely on the results from preclinical pharmacological and animal toxicity studies. In many instances, agreements on criteria for proposed pharmacological outcomes and methodology of toxicity testing are reached on a case-by-case basis. Regulatory authorities provide guidelines to outline general considerations for preclinical studies. Study design of acute toxicity, subacute and chronic toxicity, reproductive and developmental toxicity, mutagenicity, and carcinogenicity have been described in detail.[2] The major tests performed on a drug candidate during preclinical trials are shown in Table 2. These test conditions provide both the regulatory agency and the manufacturer with common acceptable procedures to achieve consistent experimental results.

1. Preclinical Development

Issues frequently arise during the planning of preclinical studies regarding the preliminary formulation of test material, selection of animal species and number, duration of toxicity studies, frequency and routes of drug administration, proposed human clinical dose in relation to animal studies, and validation of a modified test system. Usually, many discussions throughout drug evaluation occur between regulatory scientists and manufacturer in order to reach an agreement on conditions for product approval.

a. Rational Drug Design

Most drugs on the market today were developed by trial-and-error or by mass screening of natural products and synthetic compounds. These traditional approaches to drug discovery have now been modified by a more direct strategy of structure-based drug design. The important starting point is the molecular target or cell receptor in the body for

Table 2 Major Tests on a New Drug Candidate during Preclinical Research

Pharmacokinetic studies
Pharmacodynamic studies
Bioequivalence and bioavailability
Acute toxicity
Chronic toxicity
Reproductive toxicity and teratogenicity
Mutagenicity/carcinogenicity
Immunotoxicity
Local toxicity and other tests

a specific drug. The specific drug is designed to fit the target and alters its biological activity. For example, a cholesterol-lowering compound, lipitol, is designed to inhibit the catalytic site of an enzyme essential to cholesterol biosynthesis. Structure-based technology provides a means to identify promising drugs rapidly, accurately, and inexpensively. Drugs by design tend to be more effective, more specific, and less toxic than the products manufactured in traditional ways.

At the beginning of 20th century, German bacteriologist Paul Ehrlich demonstrated that drugs induced physiological effects by binding to target structures or receptors involved in normal cell functions. This type of drug would then act as a "magic bullet," attacking the target cells specifically and killing only the invading microorganisms. After the 1970s, new methods became available for obtaining pure target proteins. The three-dimensional structure of crystal protein molecules could be elucidated by computerized x-ray crystallography and imaging techniques. Progress in drug discovery proceeded rapidly thereafter.

X-ray crystallography for drug discovery was first successfully applied by scientists at the Squibb Institute for Medical Research (now Bristol-Myers Squibb) to map the structure of an enzyme closely related to human angiotensin-converting enzyme. Enzymes are favored drug targets because they control important biochemical processes. Angiotensin-converting enzyme is involved in regulating blood pressure. Using structural information, scientists could modify enzyme activity relatively easily, by introducing small molecules into their catalytic sites. This type of information was used to design the antihypertensive drug, captopril, as well as for drug discovery of targets, such as DNA and RNA, and protein receptors for hormones. Compounds designed to regulate the activity of hormone receptors, however, are more complex than enzyme inhibitors because more bonds form with hormone receptors.

Enzyme inhibitors have also been developed using the structure-based drug design method. The highly potent enzyme inhibitor of purine nucleotide phosphorylase (PNP) was developed using this technology. The inhibitor has been tested in animals for the treatment of arthritis, and a closely related compound is in clinical trials as a therapy for psoriasis and for one form of cancer. Designed enzyme blockers are useful cancer therapeutic agents since thymidilate synthase catalyzes nucleotide synthesis in cancer cells, which is essential for DNA replication and proliferation. An inhibitor prepared by Merck is being studied for treatment of glaucoma by interfering with the enzyme carbonic anhydrase. Merck is also developing another drug to treat emphysema. It inhibits human neutrophil elastase, an enzyme involved in damaging lung tissue, rheumatoid arthritis, and acute respiratory distress syndrome.[3]

b. What Is a Patent and Its Application?

Research activities in drug development are extremely expensive. A single research project can cost hundreds of thousands of dollars in laboratory reagents, facilities, investigators' time and labor, and overhead. Thus, the results obtained from drug development research need to be protected from competitors in order to foster the commercialization of unique technology into new products and maintain competitive strength in the field. Furthermore, when new products are licensed and introduced into market, the profits that form the company's main income source should be protected from slightly modified products developed by other manufacturers.

Legal methods have been used to protect scientific inventions, drug formulations, medical devices, and product brand names, including patents, trade secrets, trademarks, and copyrights. An *invention* is a new technical development or discovery in a particular scientific field. An *invention disclosure* is a written document that describes an invention. This document should include sufficient detail to permit an evaluation of:

- The scientific and technical merit of the invention
- Whether and how the invention can be protected
- Where the work that led to the invention was supported
- The invention's commercial value

The inventorship has a strict meaning. Only those who have made an independent conceptual contribution to an invention are legal inventors in the U.S. The criteria for inventorship include:

- One who first invents a new and useful process, machine, composition of matter, or other patentable matter
- When an invention involves more than one inventor, it is known as a joint invention, with the participants known as joint inventors, or co-inventors
- Unless a person contributes to the conception of the invention, that person is not an inventor

The test of inventorship is whether a person has made an original, conceptual contribution to one of the claims of the patent.

A patent is a contract between the inventor(s) and the government, granting certain rights or monopoly to inventor(s), excluding others from making, using, or selling the invention for a fixed period of time (14 years for the design; 20 years from filing date of the application). In return, the inventor makes available a detailed technical description of the invention, so that, when the patent period is expired, it may be used by other persons. Three types of patent including utility, design, and plant are granted in the U.S.

Thus, a patent encourages innovation to promote research and product development. Patents represent a unique source of technical information and an asset, which can be transferred or licensed to other organizations for financial profit. Both the institution that employed the scientists and the inventors benefit from any royalties obtained from the licensing of the invention. Patentable inventions in biotechnology include new organisms such as transgenic animals and plants, mutant organisms, such as oil-eating microorganisms, recombinant biologics and synthetic drugs, monoclonal antibodies, nucleic acid probes, medical devices and diagnostic reagents not previously developed, and novel diagnostic methods. Since enormous costs were invested in developing biotechnology products, many companies have put forth great effort in patenting their new technologies. Patents allow manufacturers the ability not only to protect their inventions and technologies from unauthorized use by competitors but also to license the products for additional financial benefits.

The criteria for patentability are defined as follows:

- Novel — the invention must be new. New uses of known processes, machines, compositions of matter, and materials are patentable.
- Useful — an invention must perform a useful function or satisfy a need.
- Unobvious — an invention must be unobvious to persons with an ordinary degree of skill in the particular field at the time of invention.
- Enabling — an invention must be described in a full, clear, and concise manner in a written patent application. The description of the invention must enable a person of skill in the relevant field to both make and use the invention.[4]

To be novel, the claimed invention should not be identical to an invention found in the prior art. For an existing enabling publication, patenting is possible as long as the patent is filed in less than 1 year after the date of the publication. Unlike laws in many countries, the U.S. law adopts the *first to invent* principle; that is, the patent will be granted to the one who proves they are the first to invent the product, even though they are not the first to file for patent.

To be unobvious, the invention process must not be something that would be obvious only to individuals skilled in the art. Sufficient technical detail must be provided in the patent application so that an individual of ordinary technical skill in the field can repeat the procedures.

The patent application consists of four parts:

1. A specification that identifies and describes the invention in detail
2. A drawing, when necessary
3. A claim that precisely defines these elements to render the invention novel and patentable
4. An oath by the inventor(s) of the invention

Generally, it takes 2 to 5 years from the initial filing date for a patent to be approved, and the anticipated cost is approximately $10,000 per case. When the patent application has been completed, it is filed with the Patent and Trademark Office (PTO). Every application filed in the PTO receives a filing date and a serial number. The examination of the application consists of a review of its compliance with the requirements for patentability and a search of the prior art, including prior U.S. patents, foreign patents, and the literature. If the invention is not considered patentable, the claims are rejected. The inventors can respond to every point of objection and criticism by the PTO in writing within 6 months from the date of mailing of the notice. The application must be amended in order to overcome the rejection. The examiner will review the response and reconsider the application. A response to a final office action must include either cancellation of claims or an appeal of the rejection. The PTO can issue a patent on only one invention described in a single application. Thus, the application must be restricted to one invention. When an application is found to be acceptable by the reviewer, a notice of acceptance will be sent to patent counsel and inventors. In some cases, two or three review cycles may be undertaken before the patent is granted. The normal duration of a patent is 20 years. In most jurisdictions in the world, the patent protection on pharmaceutical products is extended, frequently by up to 5 years, to offset the time lost between the patenting date and final approval of the drug for therapeutic use.

Scientists in academic institutions, government, and nonprofit laboratories have created an abundance of innovative ideas during the processes of drug research and development. Understanding the mechanism of laboratory-to-market procedure will facilitate the transfer of inventions to useful commercial products for the general public.

2. Animal Safety Tests

The information from animal safety tests can be used as an initial guide for comparing clinical benefits and risks for human trials. Likewise, animal toxicity studies are used to predict and characterize potential adverse effects in humans. These guidelines are intended to provide general methods of toxicological studies to appropriately evaluate drug safety and applications for drug approval. However, unified methods and routine studies cannot be expected to reveal all adverse effects of a specific drug, and it is often necessary to perform additional tests or modify the procedures of the basic guidelines.

a. Acute Toxicity Studies

Acute toxicity studies provide information about the overall profile of a drug's activity, magnitude of its toxicity, and overt effects. The studies are used to determine a single dose that will produce death in 50% of the animals. (LD50 determinations are not required to characterize the toxicity of a compound, and they may represent a misuse of animals as well.) These studies also determine any drug-induced lesion, the possible cause of mortality, and the threshold effects of a drug when given to animals as a single dose.

At least two animal species, a rodent (rat, guinea pig, mouse, hamster, gerbil) and a nonrodent (rabbit, dog, cat, or monkey), should be used in acute toxicity studies. The animal species should include those to be used in pharmacological tests, as well as in the multidose toxicity and reproduction studies. The experimental animals should be observed for at least 1 week after administration of the drug. Animals that die during the study should be necropsied.

The routes by which a drug is administered to animals should be similar to those proposed for clinical studies. Frequency of dosing by any route should be 7 days/week. The stability of the drug in the diet should be established and monitored. An appropriate number of dose levels should be used to elicit obvious toxicity or at least some demonstrable toxic symptoms.

b. Subacute and Chronic Toxicity Studies

At least one rodent and one nonrodent species should be used for multidose toxicity tests. In the case of rodents, each group should include at least 10 males and 10 females; and for nonrodents, each group should include three males and three females. When interim examinations and recovery tests are scheduled, more animals may be necessary. Subacute and chronic toxicity studies should use young animals. At least three different doses should be used: one dose level that does not cause toxic effects and a second that produces overt toxic effects. It is desirable to set the dose levels so that a dose–response relationship is achieved. In addition, a vehicle control group and/or a positive (reference drug) control group should be added.

The recommended duration of animal studies to support the Phase I, II, III, and new drug application (NDA) are as follows:

Expected Period of Clinical Use	Administration Period for Animal Studies
1–3 days	2 weeks
1 week up to 4 weeks	4–13 weeks
1 month up to 3 months	13–26 weeks
3 months or long-term repeated administration of more than 6 months	13 weeks to 52 weeks or longer

Observations and examinations should be made of the following items:

1. Gross physiological changes including body weight, and food and water intake.
2. Hematological examination — determinations for hemoglobin, hematocrit, white blood cell and differential counts, and coagulation tests. Erythrocyte, reticulocyte, and differential bone marrow counts should be made in cases of hematological abnormalities. Pretest determinations should be done in nonrodents. Periodic and terminal determinations should be done in all nonrodents and terminally in at least 10 rodents/sex/group.

3. Biochemical tests — Examinations of carbohydrate metabolism (blood glucose, etc.), liver function (serum glutamate-pyruvate transaminase [SGPT], serum glutamate-oxaloacetate transaminase [SGOT], serum alkaline phosphatase [SAP], etc.), kidney function (urinalysis for protein, glucose, electrolytes) should be performed.

4. Biopsy and necropsy — Biopsy is a useful technique for monitoring abnormal histologic status of tissues such as liver, kidney, and bone marrow. All major tissues of animals that die during the study period should be necropsied as soon as possible. Organ weights should be recorded and macroscopic and histopathological examinations of tissues should be performed.

5. Other function tests — If necessary, ECG, visual, auditory, and renal function tests should be performed.

Japanese guidelines for toxicity studies are similar to U.S. guidelines in principle and general approach; Japanese guidelines also include a more detailed description of testing items and additional criteria for specific toxicity studies. Japanese guidelines for single-dose and repeated-dose toxicity studies are listed in Table 3. Test procedures for animal toxicity studies are published by the Japanese Pharmaceutical Affairs Bureau.[5] Such procedures for animal toxicity studies are not available from the U.S. FDA.

c. Reproductive and Developmental Toxicity Studies

New drugs should be examined for toxicity in studies in which drugs are administered (I) before and during the early stages of pregnancy, (II) during the period of organogenesis, and (III) during the perinatal and lactation periods. More detailed studies should be conducted if necessary. These studies should include determination of test drug concentration in blood and tissues of dams and fetuses, or in milk, examination of drug metabolism, and direct administration of the test substance to neonates.

I. Experimental animals — Species and strains should be selected on the basis of consideration in reproductive and developmental performance, such as fertility, incidence of spontaneous malformation, and susceptibility to drugs known to affect maternal reproductive performance and development of offspring. The same animal species and strains with a low incidence of spontaneous malformation should be used in studies I, II, and III.

Table 3 Japanese Guidelines for Drug Toxicity Studies

I. Single-dose toxicity study

A. Animal species	At least two species should be used, one from rodents and the other from nonrodents other than rabbits.
B. Sex	In the case of rodents, each group should consist of at least five animals per sex. In nonrodents, each group should consist of at least two animals per sex.
C. Number of animals	Rodents; at least five animals per sex. Nonrodents; at least two animals per sex.
D. Administration route	Both oral and parenteral routes should be used, and the clinical route of administration should be included. Enforced administration should be employed for oral administration. Animals should be fasted for an appropriate period of time before the test substance is administered. When the intravenous route is proposed in humans, the use of this route alone in animal testing is acceptable.
E. Dose level	An appropriate number of dose levels should be used to establish the dose–response relationship in both rodents and nonrodents. A sufficient number of dose levels should be used in rodents to determine the approximate lethal dose. In nonrodents, sufficient dose levels should be used for the observation of overt toxic symptoms.
F. Frequency of administration	Single dose.
G. Observation	Toxic symptoms and the severity, onset, progression, and reversibility of the symptoms should be observed and recorded in relation to dose and time for 14 days. The approximate lethal dose should be estimated. Animals dying during the observation period as well as rodents surviving to the end of the period should be necropsied. Histopathologic examinations should be conducted in any organs and tissues showing macroscopic changes at necropsy.

II. Repeated-dose toxicity study

A. Animal species   At least two species should be used, one rodents and the other from nonrodents other than rabbits.

B. Sex   The same number of male and female animals should be used.

C. Number of animals   Rodents: each group should consist of at least 10 males and 10 females.
                           Nonrodents: at least three males and three females per group.

D. Administration route   The proposed clinical route of administration should be used.

E. Administration period   Administration should be performed 7 days a week:

                           Proposed Period of Clinical Use   *Administration Period for Study*

                           Single or repeated administration within 1 week   1 month
                           Repeated administration from 1 week to 4 weeks   3 months
                           Repeated administration from 1 month up to 6 months   6 months
                           Long-term repeated administration of more than 6 months   12 months

F. Dose levels   At least three different dose groups should be used: one dose level that does not cause toxic effect, and one dose level that produces overt toxic effects. It is desirable to set the dose levels so that a dose–response relationship is achieved. In addition, a vehicle control and a positive (reference drug) control group should be included.

G. Observation and examination   The following items should be observed and examined:

1. General changes including body weight, and food and water intake. General changes should be observed daily; body weight and food intake measured periodically.

Body weight: measure before the study, at least once a week for the first 3 months of drug administration, and at least once every 4 weeks thereafter.

Food intake: measure before the study, at least once a week for the first 3 months of administration, and at least once every 4 weeks thereafter.

2. Hematological examination

-- continued

Table 3 (continued)   Japanese Guidelines for Drug Toxicity Studies

For rodents, blood samples should be taken before necropsy; for nonrodents, before the study, at least once during the administration period, and before necropsy.

As many parameters as possible should be examined. These parameters include: (a) hematological examination — RBC, WBC, platelet, hemoglobin, hematocrit, and reticulocytes, prothrombin time, activated partial thromboplastin time; (b) blood chemistry examination — serum (plasma) protein, albumin, A/G ratio, protein fractions, glucose, cholesterol, triglycerides, bilirubin, urea nitrogen, creatinine, transaminases (GOT, GTP), alkaline phosphatase, electrolytes (Na, K, Cl, Ca, inorganic P), etc.

3. Urinalysis

For rodents, a fixed number of animals from each group should be analyzed at least once during the administration period; for nonrodents, urinalysis should be performed before the study and at least once during the administration period on all animals in each group.

The following items are usually examined: urinary volume, pH, protein, glucose, ketones, bilirubin, occult blood, sediments, specific gravity or osmotic pressure, and electrolytes (Na, K, etc.).

4. Eye examination

Similar to the conditions in "Urinalysis." The examination should include both macroscopic and ophthalmoscopic examinations of the anterior portion of the eye, the optic media, and the ocular fundus.

5. Other function tests

If appropriate, ECG and visual, auditory, and renal function tests should be performed.

6. Necropsy and biopsy

Dead animals found during the administration period should be necropsied as soon as possible. A macroscopic examination should be made in organs and tissues; organ weight measurements and histopathological examinations should also be performed.

All moribund animals should be killed rather than allowing them to die. Prior to sacrifice, clinical observations should be recorded and blood samples collected for hematology and blood chemistry analyses.

All survivors should be necropsied at the end of the administration period or the recovery period after taking blood samples for hematological and chemistry tests; organs and tissues should be macroscopically examined and organ weights measured. Histopathological examination should be performed on the organs and tissues of all nonrodents and of the highest dose group and the control group of rodents.

H. Recovery test

The recovery from toxic changes or the appearance of delayed toxicity should be examined in a recovery group in a 1-month or a 3-month study.

From Lee, C.J., *Development and Evaluation of Drugs from Laboratory through Licensure to Market*, CRC Press, Boca Raton, 1993. With permission.

II. Experimental methods
    A. Study of administration of the test drug before and during early stage of gestation
        1. Animals: at least one species of rodent of both sexes should be used. Species should be selected from among those used in the study during organogenesis (study II). Animals that metabolize the test drug similar to the way humans do should be used.
        2. Number of animals: each group should consist of at least 30 rats or mice and at least 12 rabbits.
        3. Administration route: the same as proposed clinical route
        4. Dose levels: at least three dose groups and a control group should be used.
        5. Control group: a negative (vehicle) control and a positive (known toxicity drug) control group should be employed.
        6. Administration period: during the period of organogenesis (segment I). The reproductive performance is divided and defined as follows:

Segment I:
In rats, days 0–7 of pregnancy
In mice, days 0–6 of pregnancy
Segment II:
In rats, days 7–17 of pregnancy
In mice, days 6–15 of pregnancy
In rabbits, days 6–18 of pregnancy
Segment III:
In rats, day 17 of pregnancy to day 21 after delivery
In mice, day 15 of pregnancy to day 21 after delivery

---

        7. Experimental procedure:
           a. All dams in each group should be examined for mortality and general signs; body weights and food intake should be measured.
           b. In the case of rodents (rats or mice), 2/3 of the dams in each group, and all dams in nonrodents (rabbits), should be necropsied at term. They should be examined for successful pregnancy and mortality of fetuses. Body weight measurement and morphological examinations should be made on live fetuses. Gross observations on organs and tissues should be conducted for dams.

      c. For rodents, the remaining 1/3 of the dams should be allowed to deliver and nurse their offspring. Dams should be examined for abnormality on delivery.

      d. Litter size, mortality, sex, and external changes of neonates should be examined. Body weights should be measured.

      e. Offspring should be examined for growth and development, appearance of specific symptoms, reproductive performance, and behavior patterns.

      f. At an appropriate time, necropsy and gross observations of organs and tissues should be conducted on treated dams. If necessary, an examination of the litters should also be done.

B. Study of administration of the test drug during the period of fetal organogenesis (segment II)

    1. Animals: at least one rodent species (e.g., rats or mice) and one nonrodent species (e.g., rabbits) should be used.

    2. Number of animals: each group should consist of at least 30 rats or mice and at least 12 rabbits.

    3. Administration route: the administration route should be the proposed clinical route.

    4. Dose levels: groups of at least three dose levels and a control group should be used.

    5. Control group: a negative (vehicle) control and a positive (known toxicity drug) control group should be employed.

    6. Administration period: during the period of organogenesis (segment II, see definition in Section A.6).

    7. Experimental procedure: as described in Section A.7.

C. Study of administration of the test drug during the perinatal and lactation periods

    1. Animals: at least one species of female rodents should be used. Species selected should be the same as those used in the organogenesis period (segment II).

    2. Number of animals: each group should consist of at least 20 rats or mice.

    3. Administration route: the administration route should be the proposed clinical route.

    4. Dose levels: groups of at least three dose levels and a control group should be employed.

    5. Control groups: the same as the conditions described in Section II.A.5.

6. Administration period: after the period of organogenesis ends, administration should be performed daily until the time of weaning.
7. Experimental procedure:
   a. All dams in each group should be examined for mortality and general signs; body weights and food intake should be measured.
   b. All dams in each group should be allowed to deliver and nurse their offspring. Dams should be examined for abnormality on delivery.
   c. Litter size, mortality, sex, and external changes of neonates should be examined. Body weights should be measured.
   d. Offspring should be examined for growth and development, appearance of specific symptoms, reproductive performance, and behavior patterns.
   e. At an appropriate time, necropsy and gross observations of organs and tissues should be conducted on treated dams. If necessary, an examination of the litters should also be done.
D. Analysis of results — summary tables and figures that give an overview of the results of all groups should be prepared. For statistical analysis of the data, the average value of the litter, rather than individual fetuses, should be used as the unit for analysis. Comparison of results of reproductive and developmental toxicity results should be made between the experimental and control (negative and positive) groups.

d. Mutagenicity Study

New drugs should be subjected to the following mutagenicity tests: (I) reversion test with bacteria, (II) chromosomal aberration test with mammalian cells in culture, and (III) micronucleus test with rodents. If necessary, other appropriate tests may also be performed.

I. Reversion test with bacteria
   A. Strains: *Salmonella typhimurium* TA 1535, TA 1537, TA 98, and TA100, and *Escherichia coli* WP2 *uvr* A should be used.
   B. Dose levels: at least five dose levels should be employed; the maximum dose of 5 mg per plate is used.
   C. Control groups: a solvent group should serve as a negative control. Authentic mutagens that require S9 mix (mixture of

nutrients and coenzyme, etc.) as well as those which do not require S9 mix should be used as positive controls.

D. Tests in the presence of S9 mix should also be performed. S9 should be prepared from the rat liver previously treated with an inducer of drug metabolizing enzymes.

E. Test methods: either a preincubation or a plate incorporation method should be used.

F. Presentation of result: the actual number and mean value of revertants should be presented in tables.

II. Chromosomal aberration test with mammalian cells in culture

A. Cells: primary or established lines of mammalian cells should be used.

B. Dose levels: at least three dose levels should be used. The highest concentration should be 10 mM or the equivalent.

C. Control groups: a solvent group should serve as a negative control. Authentic mutagens should be used as positive controls.

D. Metabolic activation: tests in the presence of S9 mix should be used.

E. Experimental procedure:

1. Chromosome specimens should be prepared twice at a proper interval after treatment with the test drug. It is possible that the treatment with the test substance may cause the prolongation of the cell cycle.

2. At least two plates should be used for each dose level. Structural chromosomal aberrations and polyploid cells on 100 metaphase cells per plate should be examined.

F. Presentation of results: the number of cells with chromosomal aberrations or frequency of chromosomal aberrations per cell should be presented in tables.

III. Micronucleus test with rodents.

A. Animals: male mice should be used.

B. Number of animals: each group should consist of at least five animals.

C. Administration route: intraperitoneal or the proposed clinical route should be used.

D. Dose levels: at least three dose groups should be used. The highest dose should cause some toxic symptoms, such as suppression of body weight.

E. Control groups: a solvent group should serve as a negative control. A drug known to induce micronuclei should be used as a positive control.

F. Frequency of administration: single or multiple doses may be administered.

G. Experimental procedure:

1. Animals should be killed 18 to 30 hours after treatment with the test drug. Smears of bone marrow should be prepared.

2. The number of micronuclei in 1000 polychromatic erythrocytes per animal should be observed and the frequency of polychromatic erythrocytes or reticulocytes per total erythrocytes calculated. Either Giemsa or acridine orange fluorescent staining method can be used.

H. Presentation of results: the number of polychromatic erythrocytes with micronuclei and the frequency of polychromatic erythrocytes per total erythrocytes should be presented in tables.

e. *Carcinogenicity Study*

Carcinogenicity studies should be conducted in the following conditions, except when a test drug is used for limited target diseases or patients and when the drug is highly beneficial to patients.

1. Carcinogenicity is suspected from the known chemical structure or pharmacological activity, and/or from the results of repeated-dose toxicity studies.

2. The proposed clinical use will extend over a long period of time.

I. Experimental animals: species and strains of animals should be selected based on the consideration of resistance to infectious disease, lifespan, spontaneous tumor incidence, and sensitivity to known carcinogens. For the same test drug, animals of the same species and strain should be used for preliminary and full-scale studies.

II. Preliminary carcinogenicity study: this study is conducted to determine the dose levels for the full-scale carcinogenicity study. If there is sufficient reliable information available, the preliminary study may be omitted; the full-scale carcinogenicity study proceeds directly.

Single-dose toxicity studies: these studies are conducted on a small number of animals in order to determine the highest dose to be used in the repeated-dose studies.

Repeated-dose toxicity studies: these studies are performed in order to determine the highest dose to be used in the full-scale carcinogenicity study.

A. Animals: at least two species of animals, such as rats, mice, and hamsters, of both sexes should be used. The study may start as soon as possible after weaning; use animals with normal growth of the same age in weeks, up to the age of 6 weeks.

B. Number of animals: each group should contain about 10 males and 10 females.

C. Administration route: the same route as the full-scale carcinogenicity study and the proposed clinical application should be used.

D. Dose levels: at least three dose groups and a control group should be employed for each sex. The highest dose should be able to cause some toxic effects. If no toxic effect occurs at the possible maximum dose, then this dose is taken as the highest dose.

E. Administration period: the administration of test drug should continue 7 days a week for 90 days. If the test drug has delayed toxicity or shows cumulative effect, a longer administration period may be necessary.

F. Experimental procedure: for all animals, the general changes should be observed daily and body weight measured at least once a week. Necropsy and gross observations of organs and tissues should be conducted on dead animals and on surviving animals at the end of the study. Histopathological examination should be performed in organs and tissues exhibiting gross changes.

G. Results: the dose in the preliminary study that inhibits body weight gain by less than 10% of the controls and causes neither death nor marked physiological changes and laboratory examination findings of the animals is the highest dose to be used in the full-scale carcinogenicity study. The highest dose should be used for each species and sex.

III. Full-scale carcinogenicity study
   A. Animals: the same condition as that described in the preliminary study.
   B. Number of animals: each group should consist of at least 50 males and 50 females. Allocation of the animals to each group should be random.

C. Administration route: the proposed clinical application route should be used.

D. Dose levels: at least three dose groups and a control group should be used for each sex.

E. Control group: a negative (vehicle or emulsifier) control and an untreated control group should be included.

F. Administration period: the administration should continue 7 days a week for a period from 24 to 30 months for rats, and from 18 to 24 months for mice and hamsters.

G. Experimental period: studies should be terminated at the end of administration; the maximum experimental period should be 30 months for rats and 24 months for mice and hamsters. When cumulative mortality reaches 75% in the lowest dose group or in the control group of either sex of animals, the survivors of that sex should be killed and the study terminated.

H. Experimental procedure:

1. All animals should be observed daily for general changes. Body weights should be measured at least once a week during the first 3 months of administration and at least once every 4 weeks thereafter.

2. Dead animals during the experimental period should be necropsied immediately. Macroscopic and histopathological examinations of organs and tissues should be conducted.

3. Animals that appear to be moribund during the experimental period should be killed and necropsied immediately. Macroscopical and histopathological examinations of organs and tissues should be conducted. At the time of sacrifice, blood samples should be taken, RBC and WBC measured, and smear specimens prepared. In cases of blood disorders such as anemia and swelling of lymph nodes, liver, and spleen, smear specimens should be examined.

4. At the end of the study, the survivors should be necropsied immediately; organs and tissues of all animals should be examined macroscopically. Histopathological examination should be conducted in organs and tissues of all animals in the highest dose group and the control. At the time of sacrifice, blood samples should be taken, RBC and WBC measured, smear specimens prepared and examined in cases of blood disorders such as anemia and swelling of lymph nodes, liver, and spleen.

3. Good Laboratory Practice Regulation and Inspection

Good laboratory practice (GLP) regulations were established in the U.S. in 1976, based on various surveys conducted by the FDA. During these surveys, it was found that many animal toxicity tests were not performed with adequate operations and methods. Thus, the experimental data could not be accepted as evidence for safety. GLP regulations were established to ensure the quality and integrity of bioresearch and animal test data submitted to the FDA.

GLP regulations are divided into three areas (Figure 3):[6,7]

■ Regulations on facilities and equipment — laboratory facilities require adequate space and structure for performing tests. Animal rooms need facilities for adjusting temperature and humidity, air ventilation, and lights. Laboratories using pathogenic microorganisms or radioactive materials need special facilities to protect the persons working in this area.

Regulations for laboratory equipment include the conditions of maintenance and management of analytical instruments and other equipment to be used in the tests. Equipment should be kept in working order.

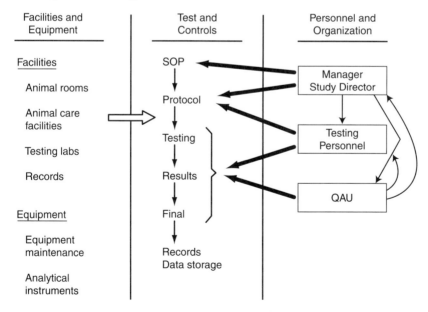

Figure 3   Outline of Good Laboratory Practice (GLP) (From Lee, C.J., *Development and Evaluation of Drugs from Laboratory through Licensure to Market*, CRC Press, Boca Raton, 1993. With permission.)

■ Regulations involved in tests and controls — for conducting animal safety tests in accurate and reproducible conditions, GLP regulations require laboratories to adhere to standard operating procedures (SOPs) in testing methods, animal care, equipment maintenance, and other areas. Protocols are designed according to SOPs for performing various tests. Test results are organized and summarized into a final report. Experimental records and data should be maintained.

■ Regulations on personnel and organization — the manager and study director supervise the planning and operation of the tests. Their main responsibilities include:
   ■ Assignment of persons to perform the tests
   ■ To monitor and supervise the process of the tests
   ■ To prepare SOPs and testing protocols
   ■ To assign quality assurance unit (QAU) and review their report and records

   Testing personnel perform various tests according to the protocols. They should keep test samples and raw data.

   QAU is assigned to persons who are not performing actual tests. The QAU is responsible for reviewing the overall test plan and operation, seeing that the tests are carried out according to protocol and GLP regulations, and proposing recommendations for improving testing conditions.

GLP inspection has been enforced since 1979, and up to 1988 the FDA had performed 690 inspections. The results of these inspections can be classified as follows:[8]

■ There are 68 cases classified as washout (WO) — this means that the inspection was not completed for such reasons as the manufacturers discontinued preparation of the product, or their laboratories did not perform the tests according to GLP regulations. Thirty-three cases were cancelled, and 17 were pending.

■ There are 572 cases classified into several categories:
   ■ 284 cases were classified as no-action indicated (NAI), which means these laboratories acted according to GLP regulations.
   ■ 20 cases were classified as voluntary action indicated (VAI)-1, which means the objectionable conditions were corrected during the inspection. These laboratories required regular routine inspections.
   ■ 141 cases were VAI-2, which means that the objectionable conditions were not corrected during the inspection, but the

conditions had minimal effect on the integrity and reliability of the safety studies.

- 93 cases were VAI-3, which means the objectionable conditions were serious. If these conditions were not corrected, they could result in official action such as disqualification of the laboratory or rejection of the test results. These laboratories needed additional inspections later.

  Among the VAI cases, 16 laboratories were listed as VAI. This classification was done before the VAI category was divided into three levels; most would be reclassified as VAI-3 under current criteria.

- There were 11 laboratories classified as official action indicated (OAI), which means the conditions were such that regulatory or administrative sanctions would be recommended. Among these, seven laboratories had their test studies rejected.

Main problems or deficiencies in meeting GLP requirements are shown in Table 4. More than two thirds of the laboratories inspected had deficiencies in one or more of the requirements of 11 major GLP regulations. The most common problem found during the inspection was the item of SOP; among 572 cases of inspection, 41% had deficiency in SOP. Forty percent of cases showed some problems in the protocol and conduct of their studies. Other problems or deficiencies included final report, QAU operation, personnel management,

Table 4   Main Deficiencies in Meeting GLP Requirements

Deficiencies	# Labs	% of 572 Inspections
1. Standard operating procedures (SOP)	235	41.1
2. Protocol and conduct	231	40.4
3. Final report	161	28.1
4. QAU operations	155	27.1
5. Personnel, management, study director	138	24.1
6. Equipment maintenance, calibration	135	23.6
7. Test and control articles	115	20.1
8. Animal care	102	17.8
9. Records	102	17.8
10. Animal testing facilities	63	11.0
11. Refusal	7	1.2

From Lee, C.J., *Development and Evaluation of Drugs from Laboratory through Licensure to Market*, CRC Press, Boca Raton, 1993. With permission.

quality of the study director, maintenance and calibration of equipment, animal care, and record keeping.

Since the GLP regulations were published in 1978, several changes were proposed. These changes imposed significant impacts in certain areas of laboratory operations and testing procedures. The main revisions in the regulations include:

1. Changes in the frequency and type of in-process inspections performed by QAU. The previous regulations required the QAU to inspect each phase of each study at 3-month intervals. However, many cases involve routine, repetitive study phases. The new regulation requires that only important phases of the study are necessary for inspection at intervals adequate to ensure the integrity and reliability of the study. There is no fixed time interval for QAU inspections.

2. The stability and chemical analyses of the testing product can be performed after the product reaches the marketplace. The previous regulations required that the identification, potency, chemical purity, and composition of testing samples should be conducted before a nonclinical laboratory study starts. Such chemical analyses are costly and take a long time. In many cases, the test product might not reach the marketplace, due to high toxicity observed in the early stage of safety tests. Thus, the revised regulations allow the chemical analyses of components and purity to be conducted after initial toxicity results are available. Similarly, the stability of a test product needs to be analyzed only for the testing period. The long-term stability study can be performed when the product reaches the market.

3. Multiple routine protocols can be arranged into a single protocol. Previous regulations required that preparation, review, and approval of a protocol was needed for each study. That is, every experiment of a test needed a specific protocol. The revised regulations allow the testing of several similar experiments under one protocol. The same protocol can cover many experiments with several test articles.

4. Changes in animal care. The previous regulations required laboratories to set up separate rooms for the diagnosis, isolation, treatment, and quarantine of laboratory animals. In many cases, a separate room is unnecessary, since the sick animals are removed or killed promptly. The revised regulations specify that laboratories need only to provide isolated rooms for specific

study objectives, such as special surgery or use of pathogenic microorganisms for the tests.

5. Changes in retention of study specimens. The previous regulations required all specimens used in the animal study to be retained for 5 years or more. However, many specimens are relatively unstable and take up storage space. It is realized that certain specimens are more important for safety evaluation of new drugs or products than are other specimens. Thus, the revised regulations allow the specimens of blood, urine, and other body fluids to be discarded after the test.

6. For identification of animals, incision of (or punching a hole in) the ear, tattooing, and other operations that may harm animals are prohibited. Coded digital amputation on animals is considered inhumane and ethically unjustifiable. Identification of animals can be achieved by marking them with pigments.

These GLP regulations and revisions were published in the *Federal Register*: December 22, 1978 (effective 6/20/79), September 4, 1987 (effective 10/5/87), and April 20, 1989 (effective 5/22/89).

When the GLP program was designed in 1976, the FDA considered only the inspections of laboratories in the U.S. and did not consider problems in other countries. Later, the FDA recognized that many drug safety tests were performed in foreign countries. In 1976, 42% of animal safety tests were conducted in foreign countries, and 36% of the laboratories existed outside of the U.S. Thus, the FDA realized it was necessary to include the laboratories in foreign countries in GLP inspection programs. If the animal safety tests conducted in foreign countries followed GLP regulations and passed inspection, the FDA could accept these test results.

Since the inspection of foreign laboratories was initiated in 1977, among 111 institutes located in foreign countries, FDA has inspected half. FDA inspectors performed GLP inspections in most laboratories in Europe, Japan, Taiwan, and Australia. The inspectors obtained the impression that these laboratories made great efforts to follow GLP regulations. Furthermore, the deficiencies or problems observed in foreign laboratories were similar to those found in the U.S. In foreign laboratories, the main deficiencies or problems in meeting GLP regulations were found in the following areas: (1) inadequate SOPs or no SOP in many operations and maintenance; (2) difference between the experimental raw data and the final report; (3) inadequate records on the change of protocols and experimental results; and (4) inadequate storage of records and raw data.

The FDA has encouraged the cooperation of GLP programs with foreign countries. The FDA can accept GLP programs of foreign countries that are similar to the U.S. program. During the past several years, the FDA has arranged agreements in regulatory activities with several foreign governments. These agreements have been developed in two phases:

- Phase I provides for a period of time during which countries develop compatible GLP programs.
- Phase II provides for the mutual acceptance of test data and affords reciprocal recognition of each country's GLP program.

Recently, the FDA has reached Phase I agreement with the governments of Canada, Sweden, West Germany, and Japan. Furthermore, Phase II agreement has been reached with the United Kingdom, The Netherlands, Italy, and Switzerland. Japanese health administration has discussed the Phase II cooperation of the GLP program with the FDA, and is expected to reach agreement on acceptance of a mutual GLP program soon. All participating countries will get mutual benefits from such cooperation and agreement that animal safety tests need not be repeated.

The FDA conducts a regular meeting to discuss various problems on present and future GLP regulations and inspections. The meeting provides an opportunity for people to exchange their opinions and information, to discuss problems, and try to find practical solutions. Hopefully, through these continuous efforts, GLP programs will serve important functions in quality assurance of the safety tests and ensure the quality, safety, and efficacy of new drugs and biological products.

Usually, GLP inspection is conducted every 2 years to make sure that the animal safety tests follow the GLP regulations, and the experimental conditions and results are accurate and reliable as evidence for safety evaluation. When serious adverse reactions related to drugs and biological products occur, a special inspection is scheduled to examine the causes of the incident. GLP inspection is usually performed by two inspectors; one person is familiar with scientific aspects and another has extensive knowledge of regulations. With this combined training and experience, this team can accomplish the inspection in a limited time.

Regulatory agencies will inform manufacturers the scheduled date, facilities, and audit items for inspection, at least 1 week before the inspection. It is necessary that the responsible persons should be present at the time of inspection to explain operating situations and to answer questions raised by the inspectors.

Before conducting the inspection, inspectors need to review various background materials, including past inspection reports, agreements submitted by manufacturers at the time of license application regarding manufacturing procedures and facilities, and pending license amendments. An organization chart describing the organization system, personnel and their responsibilities, maps of the building and facilities, as well as environmental factors that could affect animal care and safety test conditions will help to facilitate inspections.

The GLP inspection consists of two types of procedures — a general inspection, to examine the organization and personnel (software aspect), and facilities, equipment, and testing conditions (hardware aspect), and a study audit to review SOPs, test results, raw data, and record keeping, etc. If necessary, inspectors can request certain specimens, test results, or related information during the course of the inspection, and reanalyze these samples and results later. At the end of the inspection, management and technical persons meet with inspectors for discussions and an exchange of views regarding the inspection findings.

Following the inspection, a checklist helps to examine whether the test facility has an adequate operating system to ensure that safety studies are conducted according to GLP regulations:

I. Organization and personnel
    A. Obtain an up-to-date organization chart and check the relationship between the GLP testing laboratory and the quality assurance unit (QAU)
    B. Check the qualifications of the study director, testing personnel, and QAU staff
    C. Check how work responsibilities are assigned. Is there sufficient staff to perform the required work? What major changes have occurred in organization and key personnel?
    D. Check the systems for professional training and record keeping
II. Quality assurance unit (QAU)
    A. Check the systems for reviewing and monitoring safety studies; determine whether the studies are conducted in accordance with the GLP standard. Check QAU report and recommendations submitted to the study director or management.

    B. Audit reports and items inspected by QAU in the following areas:
      1. Preparation and adherence to standard operating procedures (SOPs)
      2. Regular and special inspections conducted by QAU during various phases of the test
      3. Whether the final report of studies was adequately reviewed by QAU — the report should be written clearly and accurately

III. Facilities and equipment
    A. Check whether the size and design of testing facilities are suited to the purpose of various tests.
    B. Check the possibility of contamination in the following areas:
      1. Air-flow system in the container filling room and sterility testing laboratory. What is the difference in air flow between inside and outside of the room?
      2. What are the specification limits for testing and conductivity of the distilled water and water for injection?
      3. Isolated rooms for animals.
    C. Check environmental control and monitoring procedures in the following areas:
      1. Animal rooms and areas for animal supplies
      2. Storage rooms for testing samples and products
      3. Laboratories for chemical and sterility tests
      4. Special laboratories for using isotopes and pathogenic bacteria
    D. Check that the equipment is properly located, maintained, and cleaned.
    E. Check that SOPs on the methods for maintenance and calibration of equipment are adequate. Review the records of malfunction and remedial action of equipment and check the impact of malfunction on the study.

IV. Standard operating procedures (SOPs)
    A. Check whether SOPs are available in testing laboratories and working area.
    B. Check whether adequate SOPs are maintained in the following fields:
      1. Testing specifications, storage conditions, receiving and distributing procedures of materials and chemical agents
      2. Maintenance and calibration of equipment

3. Animal care, facility, and handling of moribund or dead animals
4. Methods for testing and assay
5. Pathological and histological examinations
6. Storage of data and specimens

C. Check that all SOPs and their revisions are approved and dated

V. Animal care

A. Check the procedures of receipt, examination, quarantine, isolation of animals, and handling of sick and dead animals.

B. Check the identification methods for individual animals and cages. Is there possibility of mixing animals?

C. Check the cleaning procedures of animal rooms, cages, and storage conditions of animal care facilities. Is there an adequate control system of room temperature, light, and humidity?

D. Check the management and storage of animal feed.

E. Check for possible contamination of chemicals that might interfere with animal studies, such as insecticides and detergents.

VI. Audit on testing records

A. Check that tests are performed according to protocols or SOPs.

B. Check that raw data and records are appropriately stored. Are there possible factors that might affect test results? Check the accuracy and reliability of data and records.

C. Check the location of the facilities' archives and the procedures for accessing the archives.

VII. Final report and records

A. Check whether the final report is described accurately and clearly according to GLP regulations; signature of a responsible head and date should be listed.

B. Check whether the conclusions in the final report are in agreement with experimental data.

Inspection results are classified as follows:

I. U.S. FDA

A. No action indicated (NAI) — laboratories acted according to GLP regulations

B. Voluntary action indicated (VAI)

VAI-1 — objectionable conditions were corrected during the inspection

VAI-2 — objectionable conditions were not corrected during the inspection, but the conditions had minimal effect on the integrity and reliability of the safety studies

VAI-3 — objectionable conditions were serious. If these conditions were not corrected, they could result in official action such as disqualification of the laboratory or rejection of test results

C. Official action indicated (OAI) – objectionable conditions were such that regulatory or administrative sanctions would be recommended

II. Japanese Ministry of Health and Welfare[8]

The results of the GLP inspection are reviewed by the GLP Evaluation Committee, composed of experts from the Pharmaceutical Affairs Bureau, National Institute of Health, and National Institute of Preventive Hygiene. Inspection results are evaluated at three grades:

A. Evaluation grade A: follow and pass GLP regulations.

B. Evaluation grade B: partially follow GLP regulations. Certain objectionable conditions should be corrected or improved. These conditions exert limited and permissible effects on the accuracy and reliability of the tests.

C. Evaluation grade C: all or partial conditions do not pass GLP regulations. GLP tests performed by these facilities and conditions are not accurate and reliable. The manufacturer may submit a report regarding the correction of objectionable conditions and related documents. The Evaluation Committee will review the resubmitted report and documents to make the final conclusion.

4. Assessment of Pharmacological Activities

Pharmacology is a study of the activities of drugs and how they interact with the body. A pharmacokinetic (PK) study is conducted to establish the parameters for drug actions and to examine how the drug affects biological function. The processes that relate to the fate of a drug in the body involve absorption (A), distribution (D), metabolism (M), and excretion (E). The study helps to identify any toxic effect and estimates the most appropriate method of drug administration and the optimum effective dosage for administration. Generally, ADME studies are conducted on two species, usually rats and dogs, with various dosage levels and in both male and female subjects.

Pharmacodynamics (PD) examines more specifically how the drug exerts its pharmacological effects. The study emphasizes how a drug interacts with cells or organs, drug effect and adverse reactions, and the characteristics of dose–response curves.

The information on the pharmacokinetics and pharmacodynamics of a drug in laboratory animals and humans is important for selecting dose levels and dose regimens. It is also important for the design of toxicology studies as well as in evaluating safety and extrapolating toxicological data to humans. Figure 4 shows the pharmacokinetic and pharmacodynamic processes of a drug in the human body.

a. Absorption

A drug must enter the body to exert its pharmacological activity. Absorption refers to the entry of a drug into the blood through mucous membranes, the respiratory tract, the skin, or the sites of injection. Drugs administered by intravenous injection are considered 100% available. Intramuscular and subcutaneous injections are considered highly available. However, drugs administered by the oral route must first pass through the gastrointestinal (GI) tract and then enter the portal circulation before reaching the systemic circulation. Thus, these drugs are less available. The larger the fraction of drug absorbed from the GI tract the more bioavailable the product will become. Some drugs vary greatly in their absorption, depending on the physiological

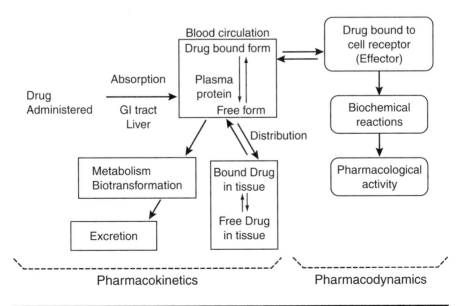

Figure 4   Pharmacokinetic and Pharmacodynamic Processes of Drugs in the Human Body

conditions. For example, many antibiotics are rapidly absorbed in the absence of food, but if taken right after a meal, the absorbed fraction is markedly decreased. The presence of antacids and chelating agents can also considerably affect the amount of drug absorbed.

There are other factors that might affect drug absorption, such as pH, certain disease states, drug interactions, and aging. Many drugs cannot be given orally because they are destroyed by the strong acid of the stomach. Proteins, such as insulin and hormones, are given only by injection. Other drugs alter the pH either by blocking the cell's acid production, e.g., proton pump inhibitors, or by acting as buffers, thus reducing the effect of the acid produced.

An important factor involved in determining body drug concentration is how much of it is bound to plasma protein. The amount of free drug concentration is directly related to the drug's activity. Thus, the drugs that bind readily to protein may require higher doses to elicit a therapeutic response. Most acidic drugs are bound to serum albumin, whereas many basic drugs bind to alpha-acid glycoprotein. Changes in the number or amount of these binding sites can alter the concentration at the receptor sites. The patient's nutritional status and age substantially affect the quantity and quality of the plasma proteins present. In elderly and malnourished patients, the plasma albumin may have less affinity for the drug, fewer binding sites available, or smaller volume of distribution. Because of these possible variations, healthy human volunteers, rather than a diseased population, are used in Phase I clinical trials.

In some cases, an acidic environment is necessary for a drug to act. For example, acid hydrolysis is necessary to convert certain prodrugs into their active form before absorption. Alternatively, an acid-catalyzed metabolism may reduce absorption. A useful form for delivery is the enteric coating that surrounds the active drug and shields it from the acidic pH of the stomach; the active drug is then released in the intestine after the enteric coating dissolves. This is the strategy behind the time-release delivery system. Various coating materials will be applied in the future for the delivery system that sends the drug directly to its site of action.

In addition, the absorbed materials from the GI tract must pass through the portal circulation before gaining access to the blood circulation. This process exposes the drugs to liver enzymes and to potential metabolism. Some drugs, e.g., oral nitrates, are removed in large portion by the hepatic first-pass metabolism. Thus, larger doses should be given orally in order to achieve therapeutic concentrations in the blood. Intestinal flora also cause changes in drug metabolism in the GI tract.

b. Distribution

Once a drug is absorbed, it should reach its target site in sufficient concentration to produce a therapeutic effect. Distribution refers to the movement of drug between the water, lipid, and protein constituents or other tissues in the body. Drug effectiveness is directly proportional to the amount of drug that is distributed to the target site and recognized by the receptor. Pharmacokinetic studies examine how much and to what extent the drug disperses throughout the body. Drug distribution is a function of the molecular properties of the product and the interaction with the biochemical reactions that drive tissue perfusion. The volume of distribution indicates the ratio of drug concentration in the body to the amount found in plasma. Drug transfer between body compartments is proportional to the amount of drug in the plasma. Drug binding to plasma protein and the quantity of water in the body compartment can significantly affect the volume of distribution.

Disease, age, and genetic defects are the most common factors that affect the sensitivity of the drug receptor, the minimal concentration of a drug to elicit a biological activity. In sensitive patients, less drug is necessary to stimulate the receptor to induce therapeutic effect. This phenomenon might be caused by the genetic modification, disease state, or other drug interaction.

c. Metabolism

Metabolism is involved with the chemical processes of biotransformation as a mechanism of detoxification or activation. Drug metabolism is a complex process involving hepatic and other enzymatic system. The liver is the main metabolic site. The kidneys, lungs, and other organs are also involved in metabolism. Many drugs form active metabolites, and thus the biological activity induced by the drug is also elicited by its metabolite. Under such situations, the activity of the administered drug is prolonged. Usually, the radioactive-labeled drugs are used to measure the metabolic pathways and formed products.

Liver function is one of the most important factors in metabolism. Several conditions drastically decrease the activity of liver enzymes and prolong the drug effect. Liver function is affected by various factors, including disease (e.g., hepatitis and alcoholism), age, drug abuse, malnutrition, and smoking. Many biochemical pathways are involved to inactivate drugs and foreign harmful materials. As a result, metabolites are more easily excreted from the body. Certain adverse reactions may result from accumulation of the drug or its metabolites in the liver and other tissues.

Orally administered drugs are absorbed from the small intestine directly through the portal system to the liver. Some drugs may be metabolized in a single passage through the liver or gastrointestinal tract. This process is referred to as *first-pass metabolism*. In most cases, the bioavailability, F, of orally absorbed drugs is lower than those given intravenously (F = 1) due to metabolism. Phase I reactions involve the biotransformation of a drug to a more polar metabolite(s) by introducing or changing the functional groups, e.g., –COOH, –OH, –NH2, –SH2, and involving enzymatic reactions, e.g., oxidation, reduction, and hydrolysis. Phase II reactions in the liver involve conjugation of the drug or Phase I metabolites with endogenous compounds such as glycine or other amino acids, glucuronic acid, and sulfate ions. The resulting conjugates are usually less active than the parent molecules. This process makes the drugs more polar and water soluble, enabling rapid excretion by the kidneys. During Phase II metabolism, if the endogenous compound is depleted, drug toxicity will occur.

Various prodrugs are prepared in order to bypass the breakdown of stomach acid or the first-pass effect. These products are biologically active compounds with their structures modified so that they maintain the inactive form and then transform into the active form through metabolism.

d. Excretion

Excretion is the removal of the drug and its metabolites from the body. Drugs are eliminated from the body mainly through the kidney and liver. However, many other organs may also be involved in the removal process. For example, some drugs cross the placenta, are secreted in breast milk, exhaled from the lungs, or excreted through perspiration.

Drugs can be filtered out in the kidney, secreted into the urine, or reabsorbed back into the blood. Renal clearance is the result of filtration through the glomeruli, secretion into the tubules, and reabsorption from the tubules. The rate of renal elimination depends on the renal blood flow, protein-binding capacity, and the physicochemical properties of the drug molecules. Lipid-soluble drugs after filtration into the renal tubules are often reabsorbed back to the bloodstream, depending on their ionization constants. Thus, metabolism assists renal excretion by making drugs more polar and water soluble. Changing the urinary pH can help the elimination of weak acids or bases. Sodium bicarbonate changes urinary pH to alkaline and helps to eliminate weak acids, e.g., aspirin. In contrast, acidifying the urine helps to eliminate weak bases, e.g., amphetamine.

Kidney dysfunction can result in decreased drug elimination and consequent toxicity. In the reduced states of cardiac output, aging, and disease, glomerular filtration rate (GFR) and tubular secretion are reduced, resulting in higher serum drug concentration. Renal clearance can be accurately measured by collecting 24-hour urine samples to determine the creatinine content. In clinical laboratory testing, creatinine clearance (CLcl) is partially determined by the measurement of the serum creatinine level. Creatinine clearance is a more sensitive indicator of kidney function than using only the serum creatinine level. In contrast, tubular secretion and reabsorption are determined through the use of chemical markers, such as benzyl-penicillin and ceftizoxime, to assess anionic tubular secretion, whereas cimetidine and ranitidine are used to assess cationic tubular secretion. Drug half-life, which indicates the amount of time required to remove 50% of the drug from the body, is commonly used to express a new drug's elimination rate.[9]

Drugs, which are distributed to the bile, are secreted into the small intestine and then reabsorbed. Biliary excretion often involves drugs and conjugates of metabolites with large molecules. Excretion of drugs through the saliva is used as a noninvasive monitoring of drug concentrations in the body. Physicochemical properties of drugs and physiological conditions play an important role in determining the extent of drug elimination through extrarenal routes.

Protein drugs are catabolized by proteolytic enzymes into amino acid fragments and reutilized in the synthesis of endogenous proteins. Their end-products of metabolism are not considered to be a safety issue. This is in contrast with the chemical drugs, which can form potentially toxic metabolites. After glomerular filtration, protein drugs are actively reabsorbed by the proximal tubules through endocytosis and then hydrolyzed within the cell to peptide fragments and amino acids and returned to the blood circulation. As a result, only small amounts of intact protein are detected in the urine.

Endocytosis and uptake of protein drugs into target organs are receptor mediated. Proteins are also distributed into tissues in more nonspecific ways. For chemical drugs, there is a direct relationship between the plasma drug concentration and the pharmacological effect. Pharmacokinetic models are widely used to describe and predict the time course of the drug in plasma and tissues. However, for peptides and proteins, there is no direct relationship between plasma drug levels and biological effect. The relationship can be described by more complicated combined PK/PD models, including PK/PD link models and complex PK/PD models.[10]

The binding of drugs to plasma proteins can influence both their distribution and elimination, and consequently their pharmacological activity. For chemical drugs and small peptides, it is generally considered that only the free molecules can pass through membranes. Therefore, the distribution and elimination clearance of total drug are usually smaller than those of free drug. The drug activity is more closely related to the free drug concentration than to the total plasma concentration. For large protein drugs such as insulin-like growth factor, tissue plasminogen activator (t-PA), growth hormone, and DNase, however, plasma binding proteins may act as facilitators of cellular uptake processes for protein drugs to interact with receptors. As a result, the amount of bound drug directly influences its pharmacodynamics. For example, growth hormone–binding proteins (GHBPs) have been identified in plasma with high and low binding affinities for GH. GHBP binds about 40 to 50% of circulating GH at low concentration of 5 ng/ml. At higher blood GH levels, the binding proteins become saturated. The clearance of bound GH is about tenfold slower than that of free GH. Consequently, the binding proteins prolong the elimination of GH and enhance its activity. On the other hand, plasma binding of GH prevents access of free GH to its receptors, resulting in a decrease of its activity.[11,12]

Prediction of the rate and extent of oral absorption of drugs in humans is important in drug development. In some cases, the rat model is a suitable animal model for predicting the extent of oral absorption in humans. Drug stability and GI absorption may differ depending on whether a drug is formulated as a solution, suspension, or other rapid-release dosage form. Absorption also depends on the dosage given. The nonlinear extent between the human and the rat can be extrapolated by normalizing doses according to body surface area and body weight. In contrast, several drugs showed much better absorption in dogs than in humans; marked differences in the nonlinear absorption profiles between the two species were found for some drugs. Some drugs also had much longer Tmax values and more prolonged absorption in humans than in dogs. Oral absorption data obtained from experimental dogs, therefore, should be confirmed in another animal species.[13–15]

5. Physicochemical Characterization and Stability

In a search for new drug candidates, researchers in the pharmaceutical industry synthesize new compounds, modify existing ones, and extract different compounds from natural sources. These drug candidates are subjected to a screening process that might involve pharmacological, toxicity, and biochemical analyses. The substances that pass through these screens are scaled up to mass production. The active raw materials, synthetic intermediates, the drug substance, and the final formulated product are analyzed for physicochemical characterization, including identity, strength, quality, purity, and stability. The information from these studies is used to identify potential safety problems in the product, to meet the requirements of regulatory agencies, and to serve as a basis for establishing quality controls and specifications for the product.

Specifications provide limits for contamination as well as accuracy and reliability of the assay. These specifications ensure uniformity of physicochemical properties from batch to batch — acceptable limits are defined for individual impurities and for the total quantity of drug-associated impurities. From a regulatory aspect, impurities can be classified as either major — an amount equal to or greater than 0.5% (w/w) of an active material, such as protein or nucleic acid contamination, which cannot be practically purified further in biological products; or minor — amounts consistently present at less than 0.5%, such as metal ions in chemical agents. Impurities found in clinical batches should be identified. A total impurity level of 2.0% has been adopted as a general or upper limit for bulk pharmaceutical chemicals.[16]

The identification of impurities and degradation products requires the extensive use of separations followed by qualitative analysis of the isolated product. Chromatographic analyses including gas (GC), high performance liquid chromatography (HPLC), thin layer chromatography, and older techniques such as solvent extraction, fractional distillation, or crystallization, are frequently used to separate trace impurities. Modern spectral methods of analysis, such as elemental analysis, nuclear magnetic resonance (NMR) spectroscopy, infrared spectroscopy, and mass spectroscopy (MS) — especially GC/MS — are used exclusively for identification of unknown products.

In addition to identification of degradation products, it is necessary to measure the rates of degradation of the drug and its formulated product under various conditions. During the preclinical animal studies and Phase I clinical trial, the short-term stability characteristics of an investigational new drug should be determined. The data provided should demonstrate that the bulk drug is stable under the duration and condition used in animal safety studies and clinical trials. In the Phase II clinical trial, the compatibility between the drug substance and other components of the final formulation system is studied.

Stability data are used to support the proposed expiration date and storage conditions that will assure potency and safety throughout the expected shelf life of the product.[17–19] To establish the expiration dating period, samples of several production lots in their market package are placed in the storage conditions for longer than the full length of the expiration dating period. The lots used for stability tests should comply with the specifications for the product in its market package. Stability tests are conducted on at least three batches of the drug. These batches are manufactured by the procedures to be used for the bulk material of the proposed marketing product. The tests should determine the effects of temperature (usually three temperatures), light, oxygen, pH, and humidity on the drug product. New stability data will be necessary when there is a significant change in formulation and manufacturing process.

Analytical methods should directly detect and quantify impurities and degradants in the products. Valid assay methods with adequate sensitivity, specificity, and accuracy should be used. For example, gas chromatography, HPLC, spectrophotometric, titrimetric, and electro-chemical methods are all capable of adequate sensitivity and precision. In many cases, quantitative analysis of drugs requires the use of an analytical reference standard. A reference standard is required when-ever a relative technique, such as spectrophotometry or fluorometry, is used for the analysis. Standards are also required for some qualitative tests such as identification by retention time, retention volume, or Rf value. The purity value of the standard must be derived from absolute methods, e.g., titrations, elemental analysis, NMR, and differential scanning calorimetry.

For pharmaceutical analyses and tests of official substances, the U.S. Pharmacopoeia (USP) and National Formulary (NF) are, of course, given primary consideration. There are several other practical and useful references.[20–23]

B. Drug Testing in People — Clinical Trials

Drug development begins with discovery and identification of poten-tially useful compounds through preclinical research. Clinical trials are the most critical steps in the process of drug development and evaluation. Among hundreds and thousands of isolated or synthesized chemicals, many compounds that look interesting in preclinical studies do not make it to clinical trials. They either lack specific pharmacological activity, are highly toxic, are difficult to produce on a large scale, or are of limited usefulness due to the high cost of development. Experimental drugs that do show promise in preclinical studies face extensive, strict, and thorough clinical trials in healthy volunteers and in high-risk populations. Usually only 1 of every 20 compounds tested in clinical trials will be found sufficiently safe and effective to receive FDA approval for marketing.[24] According to the Pharmaceutical Research and Manufacturers of America (PhRMA) a drug requires an average of 12 years and costs over $270 million to undergo preclinical testing, clinical trials, and evaluation before it can be marketed to the public.

Before a drug can be studied in humans, the manufacturer must submit an investigational new drug (IND) application to the FDA. The FDA helps to ensure that the welfare of participants in clinical studies is protected, trials are planned and conducted by qualified investigators, and that the study design and analytical method are adequate to demonstrate safety and efficacy. Without an IND application, a proposed clinical trial cannot proceed.[25,26] Pharmaceutical companies, academic investigators, or other federal agencies may function as the sponsor of an IND.

1. Investigational New Drug (IND) Application

An investigational new drug is a pharmaceutical product that has not yet been shown to be safe and effective in humans, but has been preliminarily tested in animals for safety and effectiveness. In the U.S., to formally request permission to conduct clinical trials of the drug in humans, a sponsor submits an IND application to the FDA. After a 30-day IND-review period, the FDA informs the sponsor if the proposed clinical trial is allowed to proceed. Phase I studies are placed on clinical hold primarily for safety reasons, while Phase II and III studies can be stopped for safety or design concerns. The sponsor may not start the trial until clinical hold issues are addressed. If the investigator is someone other than the sponsor, a copy of the investigator's brochure is submitted as part of the IND. An investigator's brochure contains the following information:

- A brief description of the drug substance and formulation, including both active and inactive ingredients, quantitative composition of the drug, and source of the new drug
- A summary of the pharmacologic and toxicological effects of the drug in animals, the pharmacokinetics and biologic disposition of the drug, and the information related to safety and effectiveness in humans obtained from previous clinical studies in the U.S. and abroad
- Chemical and manufacturing information, scientific training and experience of investigators, as well as information related to possible risks and adverse effects to be anticipated

The sponsor should also submit a protocol to describe in detail how the clinical trials will be conducted — the number of people participating, criteria for their selection, the place and investigators involved in trials, as well as how the drug's safety and effectiveness will be evaluated.

a. Clinical Trial Design

The optimal design for a clinical trial is a double-blind, randomized controlled study. This design provides the greatest assurance that variables possibly affecting disease risk are balanced and avoids potential bias in the assessment of endpoints. The design also maximizes the chance that a difference in disease incidence between two treatment groups is due to the drug's effect. Double-blind means that neither the investigator nor the participant knows the treatment assignment at the time the drug is being administered. Large-scale clinical trials frequently involve more than one facility in order to recruit enough eligible participants. A multicenter trial allows quicker subject enrollment and greater diversity among the study population. The choice of control depends on a number of factors, including preference by the approving regulatory authority. A "placebo" control denotes the use of a comparison group that is given a "drug" which is identical in appearance and constituents, but which does not include the active components under investigation. A placebo with similar features allows for maintenance of blinding. An active control is a comparator drug indicated for the same disease, which in most cases is an existing approved drug. Established efficacy for the relevant indication has already been previously evaluated for the active control, and similar effectiveness observed in the control group is expected when planning a Phase III trial.

For many years, pharmaceutical companies directly recruited clinical investigators to implement the clinical trials, medical monitors to ensure accurate collection of experimental results, and statisticians to analyze the data. Consequently, the pharmaceutical industry naturally wanted a return on its investment as rapidly as possible. As a contemporary solution to reduce overall cost, some of the responsibilities for data acquisition are performed by a contract research organization (CRO). Since a CRO functions independently of pharmaceutical companies, pharmaceutical companies can flexibly tailor the proportion of personnel according to the projects in hand.[27]

To protect trial participants from unnecessary suffering and respect individual rights and privacy, investigators must explain, prior to enrollment, the nature of the clinical trial and available information about the potential risks and benefits of participation. This process is called "obtaining informed consent." Patients have the right to refuse to participate or to withdraw from a trial at any time. However, because it is impossible to know in advance the possible adverse effects of an experimental drug, an institutional review board (IRB) is usually established to implement ethical guidelines. IRB members consist of professional personnel as well as patient advocates, lawyers, and consumer representatives. Phase III trials also include a data safety monitoring board (DSMB). The DSMB is formally established to review accumulating safety and efficacy data, while the trial is ongoing, for early indications of dramatic benefit or harm to a trial participant. Board members provide unbiased input, which consequently could result in premature termination of the trial.

In September 1999, a young man participated in a gene therapy trial for treatment of a rare metabolic disorder, ornithine transcarbamylase deficiency, but died due to complications caused by the investigational treatment. Shortly thereafter, more news was reported that another gene therapy researcher had not reported patient deaths in compliance with NIH rules. A federal investigation found that these investigators failed to protect the rights, safety, and welfare of research subjects, and also submitted misleading and inaccurate statements to the FDA. The deaths led to reassessment of protections for research volunteers and reminded all clinical investigators of the ethical principles underlying any clinical trial.

The concern about possible conflicts of interest has received increased attention lately.[28,29] Because close partnerships have formed between the pharmaceutical industry, academic investigators, and government agencies, personal or financial interests may interfere with official duties and professional responsibilities. Consequently, bias in the conduct of clinical studies, trial outcome, or high-level committee recommendations might occur. Everyone is accountable to ensure that data, especially from clinical trials, be scientifically robust and without ethical bias. Sometimes, informing the public about unfavorable study results places academic scientists in an awkward position. While an investigator's academic advancement depends on publishing articles, publishing unfavorable results often dissuades the pharmaceutical industry from future collaborative efforts with that investigator. On the other hand, clinical trials funded by a government agency are often perceived as an assurance of high-quality and unbiased study results.

The general public, clinical investigators, and drug manufacturers all understand that experimental drugs should be examined thoroughly yet rapidly enough that new therapeutics can be made available to patients in a timely manner. Pharmaceutical companies have an obvious incentive for accelerated clinical trial completion — the longer a trial proceeds, the more it costs. After a managed review process was initiated under the Prescription Drug User Fee Act, regulatory approval of drugs was significantly shortened. According to a 1999 report from the Tufts Center for the Study of Drug Development, the average length of clinical trials performed between 1996 and 1998 was 5.9 years, which was an improvement from an average of 7.2 years between 1993 and 1995.

Drug evaluation in human trials is unavoidable but is also the most objective method for evaluating the safety and efficacy of an experimental drug. Although these studies are expensive and take time, the process has proven essential.

b. Pre-IND Meeting between Regulatory Agency and Drug Sponsor

The FDA's Center for Drug Evaluation and Research (CDER) is responsible for the review and approval of new drug products, including prescription and nonprescription drugs. Biologic products are reviewed and approved by the Center for Biologics Evaluation and Research (CBER).

Drugs are defined as natural or synthetic substances that are effective in the prevention, treatment, or cure of disease. Biologics include viruses, therapeutic sera, toxins, antitoxins vaccines, blood and blood products, allergenic products, or similar products applicable to the prevention, treatment, or cure of diseases or injuries in humans.

Formal meetings between industry and FDA representatives can be scheduled during the pre-IND phase, end of Phase I, end of Phase

II/pre-Phase III, or prior to submitting a new drug/biologics license application (pre-NDA/BLA), or if an application is not approved.

- A pre-IND meeting is scheduled to discuss whether proposed pharmacology and/or toxicology studies would support initiation of human studies.
- An end of Phase I meeting is usually arranged for sponsors developing drugs for life-threatening diseases. Review of Phase I data and discussion of plans for Phase II studies occur at this time.
- An end of Phase II meeting is planned to discuss whether Phase II study results are sufficient to proceed with plans for Phase III trials, whether the principal trials demonstrated safety and efficacy, and whether additional information is necessary to comply with regulations for product approval. Agreements are commonly reached on the format of clinical trial reports and statistical analyses. End of Phase II meetings are particularly important for novel molecular entities proposed for important therapeutic gains, for drugs with toxicity problems, or for a marketed drug with a new indication.
- An end of Phase III or pre-NDA meeting provides an opportunity to present a general summary of the information intended to be included in the NDA, to discuss a format for the final study reports, and to resolve any major disagreements that could affect approval of the application.
- The End of the Review Conference frequently takes place after a nonapproval letter to an application is issued. The FDA and the sponsor can determine what steps are necessary to remedy the deficiencies in the application.

An opportunity to schedule meetings throughout clinical development allows greater assurance that the data submitted will be adequate, and that the documents necessary to support market approval will be provided.

2. Clinical Trials from Phase I to Phase IV

A Phase I clinical trial is directed at determining the drug's safe dosage range, the preferred route of administration, the mechanisms of absorption and distribution in the body, and possible toxicities. After initial animal testing, if no serious adverse events or toxicities are identified, a range of drug doses is evaluated in human subjects. Safety and effectiveness are assessed for a selected range of doses since animals cannot express some adverse reactions, e.g., dizziness, nausea, or pain. Likewise, human subjects might suffer serious side effects that are not apparent during animal toxicity studies. Phase I trials are normally conducted in 20 to 80 healthy volunteers and require fewer than 12 months to complete. Dose escalation in the next group of participants usually proceeds in a stepwise manner. The primary objective in Phase I studies is assessment of drug safety. Trial participants are observed closely for adverse drug reactions. Vital signs and clinical laboratory testing are also used to monitor adverse effects. Drug levels measured in the blood or tissues determine the extent of body distribution, the rate at which a therapeutic level is achieved, and the mechanism of drug elimination. All these results are used to characterize the safety profile of the drug.

Assessment of structure–activity relationship, mechanism of action in humans, and those areas in which the drugs are used as research tools to explore biologic phenomena or disease processes are also evaluated in Phase I studies. Of drugs tested in Phase I, 50 to 70% are abandoned because of problems with safety or efficacy.

The purpose of a Phase II trial is to learn more about the drug's tolerability, its therapeutic effect on a particular disease or symptom, and to select the optimal dose and dosing regimen that will be used in a Phase III trial. Common short-term side effects and risks associated with the drug are also assessed. Phase II studies are designed as randomized controlled trials and may involve high-risk populations. A prespecified primary hypothesis is stated, which traditionally proposes treatment of disease as a primary endpoint. Outcome can also be measured by a surrogate marker, such as using changes in blood pressure or cholesterol levels as indicators of the risk for coronary artery disease. Choice of the control distinguishes between natural disease remission and the effects of treatment. A placebo or the best available therapy given to the control group makes it possible to make unbiased comparisons of drug effectiveness. Studies involve no more than several hundred subjects and may take up to 2 years to complete. Approximately one third of new drugs will continue to be evaluated in a Phase III trial.

Phase III trials involve the most extensive studies to assess efficacy, safety, and optimum dose of the drug. These studies are considered pivotal, meaning that these study results provide the main information to demonstrate safety and efficacy of the drug, and provide the basis for labeling. Trials usually include several hundred to several thousand participants and are comprised of the actual target population.

Generally, two pivotal trials are needed to fulfill regulatory requirements for adequately demonstrating effectiveness of a new drug.

Sometimes, the evidence of safety and effectiveness obtained from Phase II studies is so compelling that Phase III trials are not necessary. For example, in studies on the anti-AIDS drug zidovudine, one AIDS patient died while being treated with zidovudine, compared to 19 AIDS patients given placebo. Because the results were dramatically better with zidovudine, as compared with the placebo, the FDA was able to approve the drug for marketing in March 1987 — only 4 months after receiving an application from Burroughs Wellcome.[30] On average, only about 25% of new drugs achieve successful results in Phase III trials.

After a drug is approved for marketing, surveillance for drug safety and effectiveness continues under conditions of widespread use. The sponsor continues to routinely submit adverse event information to the FDA. Since the early 1970s, the FDA has continued to monitor the safety and quality of drugs. Physicians, pharmacists, nurses, and other health-care professionals are asked to report adverse drug reactions to the FDA using a standard form, or a telephone call if the reaction is life threatening or dangerous. Phase IV studies are planned to further address concerns arising during review of prelicensure data.

An ethical dilemma involving placebo-controlled trials questions whether a control group can receive a placebo, and thus potentially be denied a proven effective treatment during a clinical trial. This dilemma is of concern especially if the proposed study population includes vulnerable populations, such as children, minorities, or participants from a developing country. Proponents of placebo controls argue that, in certain circumstances, this type of trial design is ethically justifiable when supported by sound, scientific methodological reasons and when research participants are not exposed to excessive risks of harm.

C. New Drug Application (NDA) and Biologics License Application (BLA)

After clinical trials of the new drug are completed, the manufacturer submits a new drug application (NDA) to the FDA. For biologic products, the sponsor submits a product or biologics license application (BLA). Under the Federal Food, Drug, and Cosmetic Act, all new drugs and biologics need sufficient evidence to demonstrate that the product is effective and safe before being approved for marketing and general use. Approval, however, is based on a risk-to-benefit ratio since no drug is absolutely safe; there is always some risk for developing an adverse reaction. When the benefits exceed tolerable risks, a drug is considered for approval by the FDA.

The date the FDA receives an NDA marks the start of the review process. An NDA is divided into categories, which include chemistry, pharmacology, pharmacokinetics, microbiology, clinical, and statistics sections. Upon receipt at the FDA, each NDA is assigned a submission tracking number (STN). The submitted documents are also checked for incomplete information. The application is assigned and distributed to reviewers in a specific division. If necessary, an expert consultant, selected by the FDA, can be requested to participate in the agency's review of the protocol if the study results are expected to be the primary basis for an intended indication. The FDA can also seek the advice of an advisory committee, a panel comprised of multidisciplinary experts. The review staff is required to process the NDA within 180 days, known as the regulatory review period. During the review process, the reviewers can request additional information from the sponsor. At present, an original NDA or BLA is reviewed within 6 months for priority applications and within 10 months for standard applications.[31]

A reviewer may be responsible for several NDAs at any given time; each NDA consists of numerous volumes of test data and supplements. Only about 60% of a reviewer's time is spent reviewing the actual submitted data. The remaining time is spent discussing product-related issues, preparing to testify in a congressional hearing, developing guidance documents, and reviewing the package insert for inaccurate or misleading information. The review process of an NDA is complicated and lengthy due to the need to review multiple aspects of drug development. The documents provided include preclinical and toxicology testing results, clinical trial results, description of drug composition, effect on biologic function, drug manufacturing process, and packaging.

1. Information Required to Submit an NDA or BLA

An NDA/BLA is required to contain technical information and scientific data in sufficient detail to permit the FDA to make an adequate judgment to approve or deny the application. The required technical information is as follows:[32]

I. Chemistry, manufacturing, and controls section
- Drug substance — including its physical and chemical characteristics and stability, the method of synthesis (or isolation) and purification, process controls used during manufacture and packaging. Specifications and analytic methods used in these processes should also be included.
- Drug product — a list of all components used in the manufacture; its composition; specifications and analytic methods for each component; procedures for manufacture and packaging and their in-process controls; specifications and analytic methods for identity, strength, quality, purity, and bioavailability; and stability data with proposed expiration dating.
- Environmental impact — neither the manufacturing procedures nor the product itself can cause harmful effects to the environment.

II. Nonclinical pharmacology and toxicology section; studies related to:
- Pharmacologic actions of the drug in relation to its proposed therapeutic indication; its possible adverse effects.
- Toxicological effects of the drug as they relate to the drug's intended clinical uses; the drug's acute, subacute, and chronic toxicity; carcinogenicity; and toxicities related to the drug's particular mode of administration or conditions of use.
- Effects of the drug on reproduction and on the developing fetus.
- Absorption, distribution, metabolism, and excretion of the drug in animals.

III. Human pharmacokinetics and bioavailability section
- Bioavailability and pharmacokinetic studies of the drug performed in humans include the analytic and statistical methods used in each study. These studies must be conducted in compliance with the institutional review board regulations and the informed consent regulations.
- A statement is required regarding the rationale for establishing the specification or analytic methods.
- A summary of results and discussion of these studies should be included.

IV. Microbiology section; if the drug is an anti-infective drug, the following microbiology data should be included:
- Biochemical basis of the drug's action on microbial physiology.
- Antimicrobial spectra of the drug.

- Any known mechanism of resistance to the drug.
- Laboratory methods of clinical microbiology needed for effective use of the drug.

V. Clinical data section
- Clinical pharmacology studies should include a brief comparison of clinical trial data with animal pharmacology and toxicology data.
- Controlled and/or uncontrolled clinical studies pertinent to the proposed use of the drug.
- Other data or information related to an evaluation of the safety and effectiveness of the drug.
- A summary of the benefits and risks of the drug, including a discussion of why the benefits exceed the risks under the conditions stated in the labeling.

VI. Statistical section — the statistical evaluation of clinical data

Large-scale, randomized, controlled clinical trials are particularly important because drug effectiveness can be interpreted in an unbiased manner, and the rate of less common adverse reactions can be estimated. These results accurately characterize the drug's benefit-to-risk relationship. Clinical study results are summarized in the package insert. This information is particularly helpful for physicians and pharmacists.

2. Managed Review Process

The 1993 CBER reorganization resulted in significant changes to its processes for review and approval of PLAs and establishment license applications (ELAs). During the early 1990s, PLA and ELA review time averaged 35.5 months to review six new biological products. As biological products became more complicated, testing became more complex, and the number of documents submitted in a license application increased. In order to facilitate the processes of review and approval for the development of new products, the FDA established a new policy to increase CBER's staff and resources over the next several years. In addition, CBER improved the review process for biologics to reduce review time. CBER emphasized reaching the goals of the managed review process:

- In 1997, CBER planned to review and act on 90% of priority submissions within 6 months and the standard license applications within 12 months.

- For license amendments that did not require review of clinical data and applications resubmitted following receipt of a nonap-provable letter, the review process was conducted and a response was sent within 6 months of submission.
- Meetings were arranged by the review team early in the review process to discuss whether to preliminarily accept or reject a new license application, assess the progress throughout the review period, and identify forthcoming issues for discussion at the mid-review period.
- Based on the Prescription Drug User Fee Act (PDUFA I) of 1992, CBER received funds for hiring approximately 300 additional personnel to conduct PLA and ELA review activities.

In 1997, the Prescription Drug User Fee Act (PDUFA II) was revised to include the following changes by 2002:

- The time FDA planned to review and act on 90% of priority submissions continued to be within 6 months. Standard license applications, however, would be reduced from 12 to 10 months
- Approximately 700 more personnel would be hired.
- New goals included a proposal for timeframes for scheduled meetings with industry, a mechanism for dispute resolution, and development of an infrastructure for upcoming reviews of applications submitted electronically.

The intent of PDUFA II goals was to shorten the overall drug development process. As a result of enacting PDUFA II, the percentage of applications approved increased to 80%. Due to continued successful cooperation between industry and the FDA, PDUFA was reauthorized and revised in 2002. The following provisions were made:

- Complete an initial, preliminary review of applications earlier in the review process.
- Continue to improve review efficiency and consistency between drug and biologic review processes.
- Increase surveillance of drug safety.

When the review of the application is near completion, CBER performs a prelicense inspection of the manufacturing facility described in the NDA submission. The purpose of the inspection is to verify the information and conditions described in the documents, and to examine the manufacturing process, the facility, equipment, and record keeping for compliance with good manufacturing practice (GMP) regulations. Lastly, the manufacturer's production process and control test system is visually examined. If serious deficiencies or violations are observed during the prelicense inspection, the license cannot be approved.

At the end of the review process, CBER issues an action letter to the sponsor. There are three types of action letter:

- An *approval letter* informs the applicant that the drug is approved for marketing as of the date of the letter.
- A *nonapprovable letter* indicates that the submitted information in the application is inadequate to support licensure. The letter will state the deficiencies in the application and the unresolved issues related to the product's approval.
- An *approvable letter* is issued when FDA has determined it can approve the licensure if specific additional information or material is submitted, or if specific conditions are agreed to by the applicant. FDA will frequently request that the applicant provide safety update reports and samples of the final printed labels for the product.

The sponsor has 10 days to respond to the FDA, and the response may consist of:

- Filing an amendment to the NDA or notifying the FDA that the company intends to file an amendment
- Withdrawing the NDA from consideration
- Requesting the FDA to provide an opportunity for a hearing to question the basis for denial of the NDA
- Notifying the FDA that the company agrees to an extension of the review period

During the approval process, a summary basis of approval is prepared by the FDA. It reiterates the essential findings and characteristics of the new drug, involving safety and efficacy data, pharmacokinetic parameters, and product labeling.

A supplement NDA is submitted when the manufacturer requests approval to promote an existing drug with either a new indication or new labeling, or when manufacturing procedures have changed. The review is usually less complicated and approved more quickly.

3. Good Manufacturing Practice (GMP) Regulations and Facility

Pharmaceutical manufacturers should be familiar with the principles and regulations of good manufacturing practice (GMP) and apply these to their manufacturing process. For example, the principles of GMP in relation to personnel include:

■ An adequate number of qualified, experienced personnel must be employed.
■ Personnel should have job descriptions and receive training so they can adequately conduct their duties.
■ Personal hygiene and a clean working environment should be maintained to prevent product contamination.

The principles of GMP for a facility and its equipment involve:

■ All facilities and equipment should be designed, operated, and maintained such that their functions can be carried out effectively.
■ Facilities and equipment should be arranged so as to avoid possible contamination or mix-up during the manufacturing processes of different products.
■ Sufficient storage area should be provided for materials at different stages of processing.
■ Quality control (QC) laboratories should be separated from the production area and equipped to perform their intended functions.

The facilities must meet environmental, manufacturing, and regulatory requirements, including particle monitoring and heating, ventilating and air-conditioning (HVAC) systems, water-for-injection quality, and validation programs.[33,34]

Particle monitoring and HVAC systems — The product is manufactured in a clean or aseptic environment to reduce microbial and other contaminants during the production process. Product exposure at different stages of the manufacturing process determines the class of clean room required. The classes of cleanliness are determined by the maximum number of particles ≥ 0.5 μm allowed in 1 ft^3 of air. The manufacturing processes of a biopharmaceutical plant are conducted in classes of clean rooms from 100 through 100,000 particles. The two types of areas that require separation and monitoring control are critical and controlled areas:

- Critical areas are those in which sterilized products, containers, and closures are exposed to the environment. These aseptic processing areas, such as filling and closing rooms, should be class 100 air. At the time of operation, the air should be supplied as high-efficiency particulate air (HEPA) filtered at a velocity of 90 ft/min ± 20%. The colony-forming units should be ≦ 1/10 ft^3 of space. A positive pressure of 0.05 in. H_2O should be maintained relative to adjacent, less clean areas.
- Controlled areas are those in which the unsterilized product, in-process materials, containers, and closures are prepared. These areas should be at least class 100,000 air condition with a minimum flow of 20 air changes/hour. Colony-forming units should be ≦ 25/10 ft^3 of air. Space pressurization should be maintained at 0.05 in. H_2O relative to adjacent, less clean areas.

The proposed GMPs for temperature and humidity conditions specify a temperature of 72 ± 5°F and a relative humidity of 30 to 50%. A clean room operation for aseptic filling of final containers should be maintained under positive pressure. The air flow should be unidirectional, such that materials and equipment enter the contained area by means of an airlock and leave the contained area through a separate airlock.

Water for injection (WFI) should be used when water comes in direct contact with the product, during the purification processes, media and buffer preparation, product formulation, and final rinse of glassware, stoppers, and equipment. The WFI is usually stored in and supplied to the production areas by means of a hot loop circulation system in which the water is kept at 80°C, or is passed through heat exchangers and subsequently cooled by cold loops. The WFI should meet USP or similar specifications: it contains no antimicrobial agent or other added substance, pH 5.0 to 7.0, pyrogen/endotoxin ≦ 0.25 EU/ml, total viable organisms ≦ 10 cfu/ml, nonviable particulate matter < 0.0004%, chloride ≦ 0.5 mg/l, sulfate ≦ 1.0 mg/ml, heavy metals 0.1 mg/l as Cu, ammonia 0.1 mg/l, calcium 0.1 mg/l, carbon dioxide 5.0 mg/l, oxidizable substances, pass potassium permanganate test, total solid 10 mg/l.[35,36]

The CDER has detailed regulations and guidelines defining submission requirements for new drug applications (NDA). However, CBER provides few guidelines and little guidance; it provides the form and content of BLA and facility submissions. Some aspects of information regarding the evaluation of a manufacturing facility for drugs and biological products are described as follows.

a. General Background

The applicant should submit the information that outlines the content requirements for the filing and general information including name and address of the manufacturer, location of the manufacturing plant, and the qualifications of a responsible person who is in charge of managing the establishment in all aspects related to compliance with GMP regulations.

Adequate documentation is essential for GMP. This is important for:

- Prevention of errors and/or misunderstandings described by verbal communication
- Facilitation of the monitoring of the manufacturing process of any product lot
- Ensurance of reproducibility in all aspects of manufacture

Most documentation is associated with several categories including standard operating procedures (SOPs), specifications, manufacturing procedures, and records. SOPs are required in many areas, such as:

- Maintenance and operational procedures for equipment, e.g., autoclaves, pH meters, chemical balance
- Validation for procedures such as sterilization, potency assay, and stability tests
- QC testing for procedures relating to the sampling and analyzing of raw materials and finished products
- Training personnel in professional knowledge involving manu-facturing and operational procedures

Specifications describe the qualitative and quantitative requirements or limits to which individual raw materials and final products should conform.

b. Facilities, Equipment, and Control Testing

Manufacturing formulae should indicate the product name, potency, and batch size. The processing instructions should contain manufac-turing procedures to allow personnel to undertake the process.

A manufacturer must describe in detail all buildings and areas involved in the manufacturing process, including the design and con-struction features, areas of sterile operations, and procedures for mon-itoring and prevention of product contamination.

The applicant should provide a schematic diagram of the manufacturing areas, the flow of operating personnel, raw materials, and finished products. Information related to the air and water supply systems for the manufacturing areas and animal facilities for control testing should be submitted. Furthermore, the specifications for each area of use and validation of the environment control system should be provided. The information should specify the location, animal rooms and facilities, and procedures for animal care and quarantine.

Major pieces of equipment used in the manufacturing processes should be listed and their location in the plant specified. This includes equipment used in sterilization, e.g., autoclaves, dry heat ovens, incubators, refrigerators, and freezers. In addition, the environmental control system for water and air, and the methods used for cleaning, calibrating, and validating equipment involved in the manufacturing processes should be provided.

If other products are also manufactured in the same facility, the methods used to prevent contamination and error during the manufacturing and labeling processes should be described. Monitoring systems to prevent product contamination during filling and errors in labeling should also be described in detail. It is necessary to specify the areas in which more than one product is manufactured and the location of storage and quarantine areas for intermediate and finished products.

c. Record, Personnel, and Monitoring

Through the lot number of final product, the record keeping system addresses the method of monitoring and recording the preparation of materials, production, control testing, and distribution of the final product. In cases of efficacy failure or safety problems, the manufacturer should be able to trace the production history of a particular lot. The FDA inspector might check the monitoring system of a particular product lot during the prelicense inspections and conduct routine annual inspections after the license is approved.

Many documents are now maintained in electronic format and computerized. Adequate back-up files should be retained. Also, restricted access to computerized systems is required to ensure that data are entered or amended only by authorized persons.

All personnel involved in the manufacture of drugs and biological products should have appropriate training to perform their assigned responsibilities and functions. Each individual should have the necessary knowledge and experience in manufacturing technology, and should understand the GMP regulations related to that product.

As the technology continues to improve, the manufacturing process, facilities, equipment, and key personnel will also change. Before making any significant change to major facilities, equipment, or key personnel involved in manufacturing or quality assurance, the amendments should be submitted to FDA for approval. The final products cannot be released to market until the amendments are approved.

After the product license is issued, the inspection and audit of the manufacturing facility, as well as quality control (QC) testing records, are performed periodically, usually every 2 years, by the FDA. When the establishments produce several different products, or if some products have quality assurance problems, more frequent inspections will be conducted. Many inspections are not announced. However, the FDA will notify the manufacturer prior to foreign inspections, or prior to meeting with responsible personnel for a particular stage of a manufacturing procedure. The purpose of the inspection is to ensure continued compliance with conditions or agreements specified in the PLA, BLA, and GMP regulations.

D. Postmarked Monitoring and Reporting System

The development process of a new drug or biological product does not end when it is approved or licensed by FDA — in a sense, the FDA continues to watch for problems of efficacy and safety; the process never really ends at all. Even the most extensive animal tests and clinical trials can never cover all possible conditions. Clinical trials using 2000 to 3000 people over a period of months or even a few years will not always identify a rare adverse reaction, or a probability affecting one person in a 10,000-subject population. Furthermore, drugs are tested in a limited number of high-risk populations, such as vulnerable groups of elderly persons and young children, and never among pregnant women. Therefore, not every side effect can be foreseen for the total population. For example, diethylstilbestrol, widely used during the 1950s and 1960s to prevent miscarriages, was reported to cause vaginal tumors in the daughters of the users more than 15 years later. All people involved in drug manufacture, dispensing, prescription, regulation, and use have a responsibility to reduce and prevent drug-induced disease.

An adverse drug reaction (ADR) has been defined as any response to a drug which is noxious and unintended, and which occurs at doses used in humans for prophylaxis, diagnosis, or therapy.[37] In many circumstances, the FDA approves drugs and biological products with the agreement in the form of postmarketing surveillance that continuing studies of safety and stability be carried out by manufacturers to reveal rare reactions or long-term effects. The FDA and the pharmaceutical industry closely monitor drug products on the market. Manufacturers should report to the FDA all adverse drug experiences or information they receive from any source — foreign or domestic, postmarketing studies, or reports in the scientific literature. Serious adverse reactions that are fatal, life-threatening, permanently disabling, or related to congenital anomalies or cancer, as well as unexpected reactions that are not listed in the current labeling for the drug, should be reported as soon as possible within 15 working days. Report of other reactions may be sent in quarterly or annually.[38] Approximately 1 million patients are hospitalized and about 140,000 deaths occur in the U.S. each year as a direct result of medications prescribed by physicians or those purchased over the counter in drugstores.[39]

To understand the problem of adverse reactions, the federal government has supported certain drug-monitoring programs, such as the Boston collaborative drug surveillance program and the Gainesville drug study group. The primary objectives of these programs are to detect unsuspected side effects and drug interactions, estimate known effects, and evaluate the role of influencing factors. To achieve these objectives, information on patient characteristics, drug exposure, adverse reactions, and efficacy of drug therapy should be collected. The FDA and the pharmaceutical industry have placed much greater emphasis on postmarketing surveillance of drugs. In 1985, the FDA received 37,000 ADR reports, and that number increased to 60,000 in 1986. About 80% of these reports were submitted by manufacturers who were required by regulations to keep the FDA informed of ADRs. The remaining 20% were filed by physicians and other health-care professionals.[40]

All reports on adverse reactions and efficacy failure are analyzed by computer to search for any significant patterns or clues. Results of such analyses support modifications in drug usage and regulatory action. These changes can include reduction of the dose, warning additional vulnerable groups of people, modification of the manufacturing process, or withdrawal of the product from the market either voluntarily by the manufacturer or by FDA order.

During the 1980s, adult volunteers injected with the pneumococcal vaccine manufactured by Merck Sharp & Dohme developed increases in their serum anti-A titers.[41] Later, it was reported that a platelet transfusion from a blood group O donor, immunized with a pneumo-coccal vaccine from the same manufacturer, produced a hemolytic reaction in a blood group A recipient. The elevated anti-A titers in blood group O and group B donors immunized with pneumococcal vaccine lasted for periods of up to 1 year.[42] The elevation of the anti-A titer in these group O and group B adults was considered to be due to the cross-reactivity between the pneumococcal type 14 polysac-charide in the vaccine and the blood group A substances. The structures of these two antigens are shown as follows:

$$GalNAc-(1 \rightarrow 3)\beta-Gal(1 \rightarrow 3) \text{ or } (1 \rightarrow 4)-GlcNAc$$

$$|2$$
$$|1$$

Fuc
Blood group antigen
↓

$$-6\beta D\text{-}GlcNAcp-(1 \rightarrow 3)\beta D\text{-}Galp(1 \rightarrow 4)\beta-Glcp(1 \rightarrow$$

$$|4$$
$$|1$$

βD-Galp
Type 14 pneumococcal polysaccharide

Equine anti-type 14 serum contained high levels of anti-A and induced hemolytic reactions in blood group A recipients. In addition, plague, tetanus, and diphtheria toxoids, typhoid-paratyphi A and B, and influenzae virus vaccines have been reported to contain blood group A substance. From extensive postmarket surveillance, the source of the blood group substance in these products was found to be media components in the vaccine derived from bovine or ovine tissue extracts or from chick allantoic fluid and membrane components.[43–48] Since then, Merck Sharp & Dohme has changed its manufacturing procedure to eliminate the medium component containing bovine tissue extracts. The newly formulated pneumococcal vaccine does not induce an elevation of antibodies to blood group A antigen.

Physicians usually provide adverse reaction reports directly to the Center for Drug Evaluation and Research of the FDA or to the phar-maceutical industry. The FDA is especially interested in the information of new adverse reactions not included in the drug's labeling, particularly those associated with previously reported reactions, carcinogenicity, congenital anomalies, and mortality.[49,50] These reports are important portions of postmarketing drug surveillance. The information is used to describe accurately a drug's interactions, and precautions, such as teratogenesis, toxic epidermal necrolysis, or hepatic failure for labeling. New adverse reactions are discovered more efficiently from voluntary reporting than from postmarketing studies. A report form, FDA-1639, is distributed by the FDA through the *Food and Drug Bulletin* sent to most health-care professionals. Practicing physicians, hospital pharmacists, and nurses submit more than 30,000 adverse reaction reports yearly, either directly to the FDA or to the drug manufacturer. Since these personnel are a reliable source in observing unforeseen reactions, the FDA and industry continue to encourage safety reporting by health professionals.[49,50] A better reporting system ultimately helps patients who experience adverse drug reactions. However, the voluntary reporting system cannot provide information on the incidence and rates of reaction for specific drugs. Thus, the FDA uses other forms of postmarketing surveillance, such as contracts with drug-monitoring or epidemiological studies, collaboration with the World Health Organization and other national monitoring systems, and the published literature, for additional monitoring of adverse drug reactions.

The possibility of an unknown risk factor exists with any drug, no matter how widely it is used. Although a drug has passed through a strict evaluation and approval process, a new prescription drug should always be used appropriately. A drug approved for marketing does not mean that it is absolutely safe and risk-free. The public expectation of a 100% risk-free drug could ultimately damage and slow down new drug development. The threat of lawsuits could discourage manufacturers from providing needed drugs with potential side effects.

E. Drug Evaluation Systems in Europe and Asia

1. European Regulatory System

The European Union (EU) is composed of 15 member countries with a total population of 371 million, compared to 249 million in the U.S. and 124 million in Japan, the other two major pharmaceutical groups in the world. The total European pharmaceutical market stands at £41 billion, representing approximately 33% of world drug sales. In contrast, the U.S. and Japanese represent 31% and 21%, respectively. Annual expenses for European drug research and development are estimated at about £10 billion.

During the early 1960s, the thalidomide tragedy led to the strengthening and increased legislative control of pharmaceuticals worldwide. In the U.K., the Committee on Safety of Drugs was established in 1963.

The 1968 Medicine Act established a licensing authority and created the Medicines Commission and Committee on Safety of Medicines (CSM). Similar systems of drug regulation were introduced across Europe, using external advisory committees, such as the CSM and Medicines Commission in the U.K.

The Pharmaceutical Directive was established in 1965 to create a central coordinating committee in Europe, the Committee on Proprietary Medicinal Products (CPMP), resulting in the establishment of the Multi State Licensing Procedure, the initiation of a review of older products, and requirements for the testing and regulation of all medicinal products. In 1995, the regulation of medicines throughout Europe underwent significant change with the foundation of the European Medicines Evaluation Agency (EMEA). The result is a centralized procedure in which applications for a marketing license are forwarded directly to the EMEA. In addition, a decentralized procedure based on mutual acceptance or recognition of national authority decisions is carried out by the EMEA.

The EMEA does not directly undertake evaluation of drug applications submitted to support marketing licensure. Instead, it forwards the drug applications to selected national EU regulatory agencies for appraisal. The EMEA makes a recommendation to approve or not approve the application based on the report of the national agency. Its overall role is to coordinate and manage the drug regulation system. There are approximately 140 permanent employees, and the EMEA's annual budget is about £20 million. The major objectives of the EMEA include:

- Protection of public and animal health by ensuring the efficacy, safety, and quality of drugs for human and veterinary use
- Harmonization of the European market for pharmaceutical products
- Support of European pharmaceutical manufacturing and EU industrial policy

Under the centralized procedure, drug applications are accepted for categories including biotechnology products and new chemical entities (NCEs). Approval of license applications for biotech products must be considered under the centralized procedure, whereas NCEs can be considered under either centralized or decentralized procedures. In the centralized procedure, upon receipt of an application, the EMEA staff conducts an initial appraisal within 10 days to ensure that sufficient documents are submitted. At that time a filing date is assigned. The sponsor also pays an appropriate fee (£120,000). The EMEA reviews the submitted information within 210 days. For human drugs, the application is sent directly to the CPMP for review.

Two rapporteurs are then appointed to arrange for the application to be assessed by their national regulatory authority. When the assessment is complete, the reports are presented through the rapporteurs to the CPMP. After reviewing reports, the CPMP recommends that the application be accepted or not accepted. This recommendation is then forwarded to the European Commission for its consideration within an additional 90 days. The commission usually accepts the CPMP's recommendation in making its decision. The commission has the authority to issue a marketing license; but not directly by the EMEA. The unified marketing authorization is applicable for the entire EU. It is valid for 5 years and should be renewed thereafter.

The total evaluation time for drug application is 300 days (initial review, 210 days; recommendation, 90 days). When additional information is required, the 300-day "evaluation clock" stops until the required information is provided.

In the procedure of mutual recognition, the sponsor applies for a marketing license, not to the EMEA, but to a certain national regulatory authority for assessment of the application (within 210 days). The sponsor can apply marketing licensure in other countries on the basis of mutual recognition. If one or more states refuse to grant the marketing authorization, the issues are referred back to the EMEA. The CPMP will review the problems and make a recommendation to the European Commission. The commission will make the final decision for marketing licensure.

2. Drug Approval and Regulation in Asia

a. Japan

The Japanese are the greatest consumers of drugs per capita in the world. In Japan, the manufacturing, distribution, and sale of drugs and biological products are regulated by the Ministry of Health and Welfare (Koseisho). This organization also promotes social welfare, social security, and public health. The Pharmaceutical Affairs Bureau is one of the nine bureaus under the ministry. The bureau is in charge of issues related to the efficacy, safety, and quality control of drugs, cosmetics, and medical devices. It also enforces the Pharmacists Law, the Bleeding and Blood Donor Supply Service Control Law, and the Narcotics Control Law.

The Pharmaceutical Affairs Bureau also governs factors related to manufacture, import, and sale of drugs, cosmetics, and medical devices. Its main objective is to ensure the quality, efficacy, and safety of drugs and other products, thereby promoting public health. Any company or person who wants to manufacture (or import) drugs is required to obtain a manufacturing (or import) approval and license. Similarly, any person who wants to establish a pharmacy or to sell drugs needs to obtain a license from the local prefecture government. The process of drug regulation by the Pharmaceutical Affairs Bureau is shown in Figure 5.

Drugs are classified as either ethical drugs or nonprescription drugs in Japan. Ethical drugs are prescribed only by physicians or dentists. These drugs cannot be advertised to the general public. Nonprescription drugs can be purchased directly from a pharmacy or drugstore for the purpose of self-medication.

1. Application and Evaluation for Drug Approval — The manufacturer or drug importer applies to the Ministry of Health and Welfare through the prefectural government. The new drug application is reviewed first at the specific division of the Pharmaceutical Affairs Bureau, and then forwarded to the specific subcommittee of the Central Pharmaceutical Affairs Council (CPAC), according to the type of drug. The CPAC, an advisory organization to the ministry, contains 15 committees including committees on drugs, antibiotic products, blood products, biological products, Japanese pharmacopoeia, biotechnology, etc., and 75 subcommittees. Its members consist of experts from universities, hospitals, and research institutes in medicine and pharmaceutical sciences. The council investigates and gives recommendations on important pharmaceutical and health issues (Figure 5).

New drugs are examined first by the subcommittee under the committee on drugs, according to their therapeutic category. When the examination by the subcommittee is complete, a new chemical entity may be further examined by the committee and the executive committee. For drugs containing a new chemical entity, the National Institute of Hygienic Sciences will examine its specifications and testing methods and will also test a few samples. The National Institute of Health handles antibiotics and other biological products.

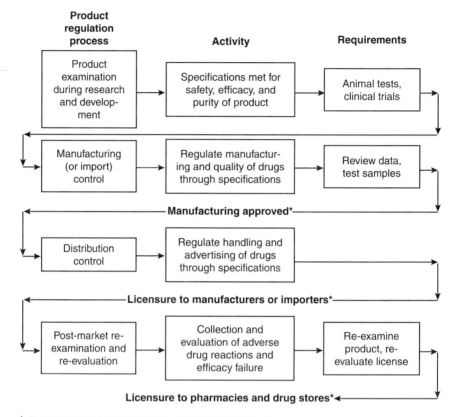

Figure 5   Drug Regulation in Japan (From Lee, C.J., *Development and Evaluation of Drugs from Laboratory through Licensure to Market*, CRC Press, Boca Raton, 1993. With permission.)

Applications for drugs containing ingredients with the same efficacy, dosage, and indications as those previously approved are not evaluated by CPAC. These applications are forwarded to the administrative offices. In general, drug review from the initial submittal of the application to final approval requires approximately 18 months for ethical drugs, 10 months for nonprescription drugs, and 6 months for "*in vitro*" diagnostic reagents.

Applications for drug manufacture or import, require the following documents or data:

- Background of the discovery, isolation, or synthesis of drugs, and conditions of use in foreign countries
- Physical and chemical characteristics, specifications, and testing methods
  - Stability – long-term storage and accelerated tests
  - Toxicity — acute, subacute, subchronic, and chronic toxicities, effects on reproduction, dependence, antigenicity, mutagenicity, carcinogenicity, and local irritation
- Pharmacological actions
  - Absorption, distribution, metabolism, and excretion — comparable data on bioequivalence
- Clinical trials

The requirements for documents or data differ depending on the nature of the drug (e.g., if the main ingredient of a drug is a new chemical entity or the same as that of a previously approved drug).

Several guidelines have been established for the preparation of a drug application:

- Toxicity test guidelines — these guidelines provide standard methods for safety tests including acute, subchronic, and chronic toxicity, reproduction, carcinogenicity, and mutagenicity.
- Good laboratory practice (GLP) guidelines — to ensure the reliability of animal safety studies, the GLP regulations were established and became effective in April 1983. Japan has maintained bilateral agreements on GLP with several foreign countries in order to promote cooperation with drug regulatory agencies in those countries, to conduct mutual GLP inspection, and to accept mutual data conforming to GLP regulations.
- Clinical evaluation guidelines — these guidelines are prepared from individual therapeutic categories to guide the conduct and evaluation of clinical trials. At present, there are 14 guidelines for conducting clinical trials for various therapeutic categories, including clinical evaluations on antihypertensive drugs, immunologic therapeutic agents against malignant tumors, antibacterial drugs, and analgesic anti-inflammatory drugs, etc. There are two legal requirements related to the clinical trials of a drug: criteria for requesting clinical trials and notification of clinical trial plans. A good clinical practice (GCP) standard was published in 1985 to provide basic conditions so that clinical trials can be properly conducted from both scientific and international ethical viewpoints.

■ Acceptance of foreign data — if animal safety, stability, and pharmacological studies and clinical trials conducted in foreign countries meet Japanese guidelines and standards, the data will be accepted. At present, however, certain clinical trials are required to be conducted in Japan due to ethnic differences in physiologic conditions. These trials include tests on absorption, distribution, metabolism, and excretion, as well as studies on the determination of dosage.

2. Postmarketing Surveillance (PMS) System — The postmarketing surveillance system includes a safety monitoring program for drugs and a policy for promoting the advancement of medicine and pharmacy. The safety monitoring program is carried out in three phases: collection of adverse drug reaction data, re-examination of drugs, and re-evaluation of drugs. Together these three processes serve as a system of checks and balances for monitoring the safety and efficacy of a drug.

a. Collection of Adverse Drug Reaction Information — The adverse drug reaction monitoring system was established in 1967 to ensure the safety of drugs. In this system, physicians and other health professionals are required to report ADR cases suspected of being previously unreported or serious adverse reactions to the Ministry of Health and Welfare. As of March 1988, there were 1049 hospitals and 2733 pharmacies designated as monitoring institutions.

During the 4 to 6 years immediately following drug approval, the manufacturer or importer of a new drug is required to conduct investigations on the use and adverse reactions of the drug and report the results to the ministry every year. The manufacturer must report adverse reaction cases within 30 days of each incidence. From the reported information, the ministry can then notify the appropriate people about adverse reactions of new drugs that were unknown at the time of approval. Since 1972, Japan has joined the WHO international drug monitoring system and reported its domestic monitoring activities on adverse drug reactions. Japan also exchanges ADR information with the U.S. FDA and with agencies in other countries.

b. Drug Re-examination — Although detailed data are submitted at the time of new drug application, there are limitations to the quality and quantity of data and information available for accurate evaluation at the time of approval and licensure. The drug re-examination system was established in 1980 to monitor the use of a new drug for 4 to 6 years following the postmarketing period. The ministry mandatorily requires the manufacturer to conduct surveys during this time to monitor the efficacy and safety of new drugs. This process is needed to ensure the drug's usefulness.

Postmarket re-examination of a drug focuses particularly on the elderly, children, and pregnant women. Usually 10,000 cases or more are used. Special attention is paid to drug complications involving hepatic, renal, blood, and other tissue disturbances. The period of re-examination for drugs with a new chemical entity, new combination, or new route of administration is 6 years after approval of the drug. Drugs with an additional indication, new dosage, or route of administration require only 4 years.

Drug re-examination begins with the pharmaceutical and chemical safety division's conducting a preliminary examination via inspection or a hearing on the contents of the drug safety and efficacy data. Then, the submitted documents are reviewed by the subcommittee and the committee on new drug re-examination and re-evaluation of CPAC. These committees in turn make recommendations on taking regulatory action. If the approval is revoked as a result of such action, the manufacture and sale of the drug is discontinued and the product withdrawn from the market immediately. The first study on prescription-event monitoring in Japan (J-PEM) was started in 1997. As of January 1989, 308 new drugs had been re-examined. To that date, there were no drug approvals revoked as a result of re-examination. The second study was conducted in 2001, supported by the Ministry of Health and Welfare. Official guidelines will be issued.[50a]

c. Drug Re-evaluation

First round re-evaluation — based on administrative guidance. The drug re-evaluation system was established in 1971. The system was proposed by the drug efficacy advisory council in response to the thalidomide tragedy during the 1960s. Between 1973 and 1989, a total of 18,986 products were re-evaluated, which included 1765 substances contained in prescription drugs. As a result, 1079 prescription drugs were determined as "having no basis for indicated usefulness." Similarly, in 1988 among 1269 combination drugs, 190 items were judged with the same conclusion. Drugs were labeled as "having no basis for indicated usefulness" for the following reasons: insufficient basis for efficacy, adverse drug reactions outweighed the therapeutic benefit, inadequate duration to achieve therapeutic drug levels, and inadequate dosage form.

Second round re-evaluation — based on Pharmaceutical Affairs Law. Drugs subjected to this re-evaluation include newly developed drugs approved after October 1, 1967, and those drugs containing the same ingredients as newly developed drugs but which were exempted from the first re-evaluation based on administrative guidance.

In the second evaluation program, 129 formulas out of 611 items have been selected for re-evaluation; one item has been judged "not useful."

New re-evaluation system — since May 1988, all prescription drugs shall be reviewed every 5 years.

The ADR Suffering Relief Fund Law was established in 1979 to provide prompt relief for sufferers of disease, disability, or death caused by adverse reactions despite proper use of drugs. The sufferers receive compensation such as reimbursement for medical expenses, damage pensions, and survivor's pensions. The fund operations are supported by drug manufacturers, importers, and government subsidies.

In 1987, this law was expanded to include the promotion of pharmaceutical research and development and technology through subsidy and loan programs. Thus, the name has been changed to the ADR Suffering Relief/Research Promotion Funds Law.

There are three basic steps in the Japanese regulatory system:

■ Approval must be obtained for manufacture or import of drugs.
■ Drug-re-examination is performed for licensure process.
■ An official drug price must be given.

The regulatory process emphasizes that at least some clinical trials be conducted in Japan, due to differences in body size and metabolism of Japanese, compared to U.S. or European people. In addition, the dosage of active ingredient contained in Japanese drugs is lower than in many areas of the world. Therefore, small-scale clinical trials should be conducted for drugs to be used in Japanese people to evaluate their efficacy and safety.

b. Taiwan

The island state of Taiwan, with a population of 23 million, has achieved an annual growth rate of approximately 10% during the decade of 1981 to 1991. According to the *World Development Report 2002 — Building Institutions for Markets,* Taiwan was the world's 16th largest economy in 2000. Taiwan's Gross National Product (GNP) was $313.9 billion and per capita GNP $14,188 in 2000, which would place

Taiwan 16th worldwide. It ranks among the highest GNPs in Asia. In 1990, the gross production of Taiwan's pharmaceutical industry reached U.S. $1.2 billion.

1. Regulatory Aspects of Drugs and Biologics — Health agencies in Taiwan are organized at four levels: national, city and province, county and city, and township. At the national level, the Department of Health (DOH) of the Executive Yuan is the highest health authority. The department has several bureaus including the Bureau of Pharmaceutical Affairs, the National Laboratories of Foods and Drugs, and the Narcotics Bureau. The department plans, supervises, assists, and coordinates health programs throughout the country.

The manufacturing, importation, and sale of medicines and medical devices are subject to inspection and registration in advance. In applying for inspection and registration, domestically manufactured drugs, including chemical and herbal medicines, must be tested for safety to ensure their quality. The manufacturers can apply for registration and market approval only when they meet cGMP (current good manufacturing practice) regulations. The application for registration of new drugs and market approval requires documentation of the free sale certificates from at least three of the ten advanced countries in new drug research and development (Germany, U.S., U.K., France, Japan, Switzerland, Canada, Australia, Belgium, and Sweden). For the new pharmaceutical ingredients approved after 1988, the generic products application for approval should be accompanied by information on the bioavailability or bioequivalence tests. Biological products, when manufactured or imported under permit licenses, can only be sold after batch-wise laboratory certification.

Local health agencies conduct regular and unscheduled inspections and sampling testings of medicines and cosmetics that are manufactured, imported, and sold in their areas. Samples are sent to the National Laboratories of Foods and Drugs for analysis to ensure safety.

To upgrade the standards of the pharmaceutical industry, the Department of Health and the Ministry of Economic Affairs jointly issued GMP regulations in 1982. By September 2002, 153 pharmaceutical factories had been approved as cGMP factories. Regular and unscheduled inspections of these factories have been conducted by the department. For non-cGMP factories, the department assists them in contracting the manufacturing of their medicines out to cGMP factories in order to allow them to stay in business.

To adequately protect the patent right of new drugs and to promote the research and development of domestic pharmaceutical industries, the department established in 1983 a safety surveillance system for new drugs. Local agents of new drugs are instructed to conduct, within 3 years, safety surveillance of their new drugs in designated teaching hospitals and to supply information on the side effects of these new drugs at any time. Domestic manufacturers that comply with cGMPs may be eligible to apply for the registration and market approval of a generic drug from the original manufacturer.

The objective of safety surveillance of new drugs is to detect any adverse effects of the drugs that have not previously been discovered in clinical trials.

b. Challenges in Development and Evaluation — The government of the Republic of China in Taiwan considers the pharmaceutical industry as one of the top priorities in its national development plan. It has realized that if a nation intends to develop its pharmaceutical industry, the ultimate goal should be an industry with the capability to produce novel proprietary drugs. Taiwan's pharmaceutical industry is facing the challenge of moving from the development of generic drugs to the technologically more advanced and high value-added products such as new formulations and new chemical entity drugs. In the transition process, the government must play a critical role in building a good working environment, including setting up adequate drug regulations, strengthening R & D capabilities, and providing investment capital. Taiwan also has to establish the competitive ability to engage in the international drug market. To achieve this objective, the government has created the Development Center for Biotechnology (DCB) to establish a pharmaceutical research and development laboratory. It coordinates clinical studies of promising new drugs for ultimate commercialization in the global market. It also assists local pharmaceutical companies to develop bulk raw materials and generic versions of off-patent drugs.

The evaluation of new drug applications (NDAs) in Taiwan was previously performed by a drug advisory committee composed of external experts invited by the Bureau of Pharmaceutical Affairs. The old system could not perform independent reviews of drug applications and required preapproval (licensed products) from major foreign governments before submission. The part-time academic advisory boards have offered little assistance to the pharmaceutical industry in regulatory drug development. In answer to the national policy of developing its pharmaceutical industry and competition in globalization of free trade, the Center for Drug Evaluation (CDE) was established as a nongovernmental, nonprofit foundation by DOH in 1998 to meet the new challenge of effective NDA reviews. CDE assists in evaluating clinical trial protocols for new drugs, herbal medicines, and biologics. At present, CDE has 43 full-time employees and plans to have 80 to 100 employees in 5 years.

Most new drugs are developed in the U.S. and Europe with very little Asian data in the clinical trials. The extrapolation of these clinical data to Asian populations has not been evaluated extensively in Asian countries. Thus, the bridging studies using Asian populations become an immediate challenge for the regulatory agencies. DOH has accepted NDAs without free sale certificates from reference countries since 2001/2002. The NDA reviews, without involving the evaluations of advanced countries, exert a new challenge for CDE in independent regulatory judgment and managing adverse drug reactions monitoring.

As a new institution, CDE has suffered some growing pains, including recruiting and retaining competent staff, keeping harmonious relationships with other agencies, and earning the trust of industry and sponsors. Furthermore, there is a lack of original applications with high-quality protocols for clinical trials to review. As the new CDE strives to meet the demand of its increasing workload, many tough challenges lie ahead.

The Asian-Pacific region represents a large and densely populated area, but is also a region with small individual markets, weak regulatory authorities, primitive local drug industries, and a poor system of conducting clinical trials. Except for Japan, the region has been excluded from the International Conference on Harmonization (ICH), has no independent voice in global drug evaluation processes, and its local need for new drug development is frequently ignored. Therefore, an independent drug review system for this region is needed to account for the population difference in drug response, to promote local industry, and to meet regional needs for new drugs.

To achieve this goal, the Asian-Pacific region should establish a unified market for new drugs to provide a favorable environment and harmonized regulatory system. It is thus considered that the regulatory agencies in the region pool their resources and collaborate on drug regulations to examine the issues related to clinical bridging studies, collaborate on inspections, share postmarket monitoring, establish joint review of new drug applications, and eventually mutual recognition of new drug approval.[51–53]

3. International Conference on Harmonization (ICH) for Standardization and Simplified Regulation

The International Conference on Harmonization (ICH) brings together the regulatory authorities of Europe, Japan, and the U.S., and experts from the pharmaceutical industries in the three regions, in order to seek ways to eliminate redundant and duplicate technical requirements for registering new drugs and biologics. The main objective is to expedite the global development and availability of new medicines without sacrificing efficacy, safety, or quality.

The six co-sponsors of the ICH include:

- Europe:
    - Commission of the European Communities (CEC)
    - European Federation of Pharmaceutical Industries' Association (EFPIA)
- Japan:
    - Ministry of Health and Welfare (MHW)
    - Japan Pharmaceutical Manufacturers Association (JPMA)
- U.S.:
    - Food and Drug Administration (FDA)
    - Pharmaceutical Research and Manufacturers of America (PhRMA)

In addition, the International Federation of Pharmaceutical Manufacturers Association (IFPMA) participates as an umbrella organization for the pharmaceutical industry and provides the ICH Secretariat.

The first meeting (ICH1) was held in Brussels in 1991, hosted by CEC and EFPIA. Representatives of the regulatory agencies and industry associations of Europe, Japan, and the U.S. met to plan an international conference to discuss issues on harmonization of safety, quality, and efficacy. ICH2 was held in Orlando, Florida, in 1993. ICH2 highlights include progress in the harmonization of clinical safety reporting requirements in clinical trials. The use of common definitions and reporting procedures reduces the potential confusion and eliminates certain duplicate practices:

- Efficacy — the guideline on the extent of population exposure emphasized that it is required to assess clinical safety for medicinal products intended for long-term treatment of non-life-threatening conditions.
- Safety — the guideline on reproductive toxicology was prepared to save research time and resources and eliminate duplicate

animal testing. The carcinogenicity testing procedures allow end-points other than maximum tolerated dose (MTD).

■ Quality — the guideline on stability testing grants assessing new molecules under a standard set of temperature and humidity conditions.

The biennial ICH meetings (Yokohama, Japan, 1995; and Brussels, Belgium, 1997) have disseminated information on ICH and ensured that harmonization is conducted in an open and transparent manner. ICH4 in 1997 marked the completion of the first phase of ICH activities toward the goal of reducing duplication in the process for developing new medicinal products and submitting technical data for registration. The second phase of ICH activities has aimed at ensuring that good quality, safe, and effective medicines are developed in the most expeditious and cost-effective manner to prevent unnecessary duplication of clinical trials in humans and to minimize the use of animals without compromising the regulatory obligations of safety and efficacy.

During ICH5 held in November 2000 in San Diego, California, the guideline "Good Manufacturing Practices for Active Pharmaceutical Ingredients" reached final consensus. The most important achievement in ICH5 was reaching final consensus on the guidelines describing a common format for pharmaceutical product submission known as the Common Technical Document (CTD). Industry will be able to use the CTD in the three ICH regions (the U.S., the European Union, and Japan), as well as the observer organizations (Canada and Switzerland). Arrangement was made to hold another large conference (ICH6) in Japan in 2003.

II. QUALITY ASSURANCE — REGULATION AND CONTROL TESTS

Quality assurance (QA) and quality control (QC) follow regulations and standard operating procedures directed toward ensuring the efficacy, safety, and purity of drug production. The FDA has issued *Current Good Manufacturing Practice for Finished Pharmaceuticals* (cGMP) and guidelines regarding manufacturing operations and assessment of product quality. These guidelines also serve as the basis for compliance and inspection of facilities and operations.

QA and QC have different functions within an organization. QC functions test and measure materials and final products. QA establishes a system for ensuring the quality of products. The QA division usually reports to the chief executive officer or the president of a company. QA is independent of the economic issues related to manufacturing and distribution of the products. It assists in identifying and preparing the required standard operating procedures (SOPs) related to quality control. It determines that the products meet all the applicable specifications and that they were manufactured following the regulations of the GMPs.

One major responsibility of QA is a quality monitoring and audit of production records to determine if manufacturing operations have adequate system, facilities, and written records for the quality evaluation of the products.

Quality control is responsible for the control testing of incoming raw materials and products, as well as inspection of packaging contents and labeling. QC scientists conduct in-process testing and environmental monitoring, and inspect operations for compliance. Their primary functions include analytical laboratory testing of products; sampling, inspection, and testing of incoming raw materials; packaging and labeling contents; checking operations at the important intermediate steps; and control of a product through its distribution.

Product specifications describing the limits for acceptance parameters should be prepared and validated on the test methods for evaluating raw material and products. QC is also responsible for monitoring the environmental conditions under which products are manufactured to determine the acceptable level of air particles and microbial contaminants. This monitoring and control of the environment will ensure the quality and stability of the product by keeping the product from being exposed to a deleterious environment.

A. FDA's Basic Concept of Regulation

Following the steps of rapid medical, pharmaceutical, and biotechnological progress, the public demand for quality health and medical services has increased. Faced with the challenge of matching supply with demand, the FDA has established a system of control and regulation of drugs and biological products.[54]

■ FDA has realized that the basic concept of enlightened regulation is to maintain an organization with strong research capability. Experience in basic medical research helps solve potential problems in the manufacture and testing of licensed drugs and investigational products. Investigators in charge of control tests should not only be familiar with analytical techniques, but should also maintain close and continual contact with products developed by the manufacturer. This scientific approach to problemsolving, rather than merely enforcing control tests, has improved cooperation with manufacturers to solve technical difficulties with drug analysis, develop more effective methods for drug evaluation, ensure the quality of products, and provide a continual supply of effective drugs and biological products. Based on this integral approach, the Bureau of Biologics was reorganized into the Center for Biologics Evaluation and Research, which carries out regulatory responsibilities and control tests of biological products. It also conducts basic research in many areas.

■ Another approach to the regulatory process is a continual consultation and exchange of opinions with the scientific community. During the process of licensure, particularly before making important regulatory decisions, representatives from the academic community, medical and pharmaceutical associations, and from other government agencies are consulted to review and discuss scientific data and issues with FDA staff and manufacturers. Many advisory committees have been established to review and make recommendations before enforcing critical decisions. Thus, the FDA's final decisions generally reflect a consensus of scientific and medical opinion. The continual cooperation and exchange of scientific information are also achieved through presentation of research data and opinions of experts in various conferences, seminars, and workshops.

B. Lot Release Specifications and Control Tests

Recently, there has been an increased emphasis on analytical chemistry involved in the processes of drug discovery, development, and manufacturing. More advanced instrumental analysis, assisted by computer, provides greater sensitivity and efficiency. These technical flows emphasize the requirement for more stability-indicating assay methods and evaluation of impurities in drug products. High performance liquid chromatography (HPLC) methods have been used widely in many laboratories. Elimination of tests that require animals is enforced by the replacement of a rabbit pyrogen test with the bacterial endotoxin method.

The use of an analytical method is justified after it has been validated. In a section of *Validation of Compendial Methods*, the USP describes analytical parameters that should be measured to validate analytical procedures. These parameters include precision (reproducibility); accuracy (exactness); limit of detection (concentration that gives the limit perceptible response); sensitivity (lowest concentration measurable with good precision and accuracy); selectivity (ability to measure in the presence of possible impurities); range and linearity (the concentration range over which concentration and response are related linearly); and ruggedness (degree of reproducibility of results in various conditions, such as different instruments, analysts, or laboratories).

Drugs may interfere with the interpretation of laboratory tests by the following mechanisms:

- Biochemical interference due to the reaction of a drug or its metabolites in biological systems to test reagents in analytical procedures. For example, the false-positive urine glucose results due to the reducing properties of drugs, such as ascorbic acid, p-aminosalicylic acid, tetracycline, or levodopa, which are excreted in urine.
- Pharmacological interference due to drug-induced alterations in various physiological conditions, such as the decrease in serum potassium levels in patients given thiazide diuretics, and the elevation in plasma proteins. Drug–drug interaction can also result in changes in these parameters. Barbiturates induce hepatic microsomal enzyme synthesis and increase the metabolism and decrease the therapeutic effect of drugs, e.g., warfarin, even after these drugs are discontinued.
- Toxicological interference as a result of toxicity of a drug. For example, changes in liver- and kidney-function tests and hematological abnormality (anemia, leukopenia) can be due to drug-induced toxicity.

The enzyme-linked immunosorbent assay (ELISA) has been widely used in immunochemical tests to detect antibodies by a technique using enzyme-linked antibodies to label antigenic substances in tissue or body fluid. The antigen is attached to a solid matrix and reacts with a specimen that may contain a complementary antibody. The anti-human immunoglobulin, which is conjugated with the enzyme, is added and the antigen reacts with the bound antibody of the patient. By adding the substrate reagent, the enzymatic reaction is measured. This test system has been used to identify antibodies to bacterial and viral products and in the quantitation of many drugs.

HPLC and gas chromatography (GC) have been extensively used because of their analytical capabilities. HPLC has been rapidly developed with the introduction of new pumping methods, more reliable columns, and a variety of detectors. The chromatographic procedure and instrumentation may be so designed that the method is automated in sampling, separation, detection, recording, calculation, and printing of results. In GC, any compound, directly or with derivatization, can be analyzed if it has a perceptible vapor pressure and if a suitable column or detector can be used.

Other widely used instruments which are applicable for routine analyses include the spectrophotometer, nephelometer (measuring antigen–antibody binding), fluorometer (measuring fluorescence that may be present in the sample), emission spectrography (for quantitative analysis of many elements), and flame atomic absorption spectrometer (for routine determination of alkali metals and alkaline earth metals).

Before distribution of drug products to the market, manufacturers must conduct control tests to ensure that the products meet specifications and lot-to-lot consistency in the quality of the product. FDA laboratories review the manufacturers' test results and perform various tests on representative lot samples, if necessary, to ensure that the licensed products continue to meet regulatory requirements.

Manufacturers must submit samples of both the purified bulk product and the final container product. The bulk product is analyzed by FDA laboratories for the identity and physicochemical characterization of the product, impurities, and other contaminants. The final product of biologics is tested for potency, identity, sterility, general safety, and pyrogenicity or endotoxin content.[54]

During the process of a lot release test, CBER/FDA has observed that the several biologic products are extremely stable under the specified manufacturing and storage conditions. Thus, it might not be necessary to test every lot sample of these stable products. Manufacturers that have demonstrated an acceptable history of lot release and quality control in the manufacturing process may submit a PLA amendment requesting lot release alternatives. However, if there are significant changes in the manufacturing procedure and facility, or if deficiencies are observed during the inspection and lot release testing, CBER reimposes the lot release requirement.

1. Control Tests for Bacterial Glycoconjugate Vaccines

Haemophilus polysaccharide (PS)-protein conjugate vaccine — Haemophilus influenzae type b (Hib) is the most common cause of bacterial meningitis in the U.S. It occurs primarily among children under 5 years of age and is responsible for other diseases, including epiglottitis, septic arthritis, osteomyelitis, pericarditis, and pneumonia. In 1985, the Hib PS vaccine was licensed for use in children over the age of 18 to 24 months. Furthermore, the Hib conjugate vaccine was approved in the U.S. (1987) for use in children 18 months and older. Produced by two manufacturers, this vaccine was approved in 1990 for immunization of infants at 2 months of age. The Hib conjugate and DTP (diphtheria, tetanus, and pertussis) combined vaccine became available in 1993. As a result, the incidence of childhood Hib diseases in the U.S. has been reduced dramatically.[55]

Although Hib conjugate vaccines from different manufacturers use the same polyribose ribitol phosphate (PRP) antigen, the chemical modifications and antigenic configurations of these vaccines are quite different. In addition, studies of the immune responses of different conjugates utilize different clinical trial designs and antibody assay conditions. Therefore, each conjugate vaccine has been tested and regulated on a case-by-case basis, resulting in different specifications for each vaccine (Table 5).

The Hib conjugate bulk concentrate and final product should meet these specifications defining the physicochemical characteristics and contamination limits determined by regulatory methods. Manufacturers usually propose analytical methods and product specifications. FDA scientists review, evaluate, make recommendations, and accept valid test methods and specifications. They do not develop the test methods for a new biological product. Instead, the FDA scientists evaluate test results submitted by the manufacturers. It is the responsibility of manufacturers to submit valid analytical methods and carry out these tests.

Pneumococcal PS and glycoconjugate vaccines — the current pneumococcal PS vaccine is composed of 23 types of purified PSs: types 1, 2, 3, 4, 5, 6B, 7F, 8, 9N, 9V, 10A, 11A, 12F, 14, 15B, 17F, 18C, 19F, 19A, 20, 22F, 23F, and 33F. It was licensed in the U.S. in 1983, replacing a 14-valent vaccine licensed in 1977. Most healthy adults, including the elderly, induce a twofold or greater rise in type-specific antibody within 2 to 3 weeks after vaccination. In children younger than 2 years of age, the antibody response to most types is generally poor. The pneumococcal vaccine has been shown to be safe and effective in preventing pneumococcal infection in young adults and elderly persons. The U.S. FDA product release specifications for pneumococcal PSs are shown in Table 6.[56] The WHO's proposed requirements for pneumococcal vaccine[57] are comparable to those of the FDA.

The specifications on the chemical content of pneumococcal PSs are established based on (a) the results of chemical analyses performed by CBER on PS samples submitted by different manufacturers, (b) the results of chemical analyses by the manufacturers, and (c) reported chemical structure of the PS from the literature. These specifications can be modified as the technology of PS preparation and analytical techniques are improved. For example, a high-field proton nuclear magnetic resonance (NMR) method has been applied for the identity of PSs. The specificity and reproducibility of the NMR-based identity

Table 5   Characteristics and Specifications for Hib Conjugate Vaccines

	Manufacturer		
	Aventis Pasteur	*Wyeth-Lederle*	*MSD*
Characteristics			
1. PS size	Heat-sized, medium	Periodate oxidized, about 20 PRP unit oligo-saccharide	Native, large PS
2. Protein carrier	Tetanus toxoid	CRM197, non-toxic variant of diphtheria toxin	Meningococcal outer membrane protein (OMP)
3. Spacer linkage or reactant	ADH	No	PS-carbamate, homocysteine
4. Conjugate reaction	CNBr activation, carbodiimide coupling	Reductive amination	Carbamate-thioester conjugation
Specifications			
Vaccine	*PRP-TT*	*HbOC*	*PRP-OMPC*
1. Polysaccharide (PRP, %)			
Ribose	≥32	≥32	35–45
Protein	≤1	≤1	≤1
Nucleic acid	≤1	≤1	≤1
Phosphorus	(%) 6.8–9.0	–	7–9
LPS (EU/μg PS)	≤10	≤1.0	–
2. Protein carrier			
	TT	*CRM197*	*MOMP*
Purity (%)	≥50	≥90	≥60
Sialic acid (%)	–	–	≤1
Nucleic acid	–	≤1	≤1

-- continued

Table 5 (continued)   Characteristics and Specifications for Hib Conjugate Vaccines

Specifications	Manufacturer		
	Aventis Pasteur	Wyeth–Lederle	MSD
Pyrogenicity (µg/ml/kg body wt)	2	≤ 1.0 EU/ ug protein	0.025
High mol. Wt. conj.	≥75%	–	–
3. Bulk concentrate			
Free ribose (%)	≤37	≤10	–
PS/protein	2.4 ± 0.6	0.30–0.70	0.05–0.10
Molecular size (Sepharose CL-2B)	≥60%, 0.2 (CL-4B)	0.3–0.6 (CL-4B)	≥85%, 0.25
LPS (EU/µg PS)	–	–	≤10
Pyrogenicity (µg/ml/kg.b.wt.)	–	1.0	0.025
4. Final container			
PS (µg/dose)	10 ± 2	10 ± 2	15 ± 3
P Ug/dose)	0.84 ± 20%	–	–
Pyrogenicity (µg/ml/kg.b.wt.)	0.1	1.0	IV, 0.025 IM, 10
LPS (EU/ml)	≤100	≤50	≤20
Free ribose (%)	–	≤10	–
Free protein	–	≤ 1	–
Mouse immunogenicity	–	–	+
Sterility	+	+	+
General safety	+	+	+
Identity	+	+	+

Abbreviations: MSD, Merck, Sharp & Dohme; PS, Polysaccharide; PRP, Polyribosylribitol phosphate; MOMP, Meningococcal group B outer membrane protein; CRM197, Diphtheria toxin mutant protein; TT, Tetanus toxoid; ADH, Adipic dihydrazide; CNBr, Cyanogen bromide; LPS, Lipopolysaccharide; EU, Endotoxin unit; kg.b.wt., Kilogram body weight; P, Phosphorus.

From Lee, C.J., *Managing Biotechnology in Drug Development*, CRC Press, Boca Raton, 1996. With permission.

assay is superior to the colorimetric assays and has been adapted for use in quality control. In addition, the NMR spectrum can be integrated to quantitate residues contained in the PS, e.g., ethanol, isopropanol, acetone, phenol, acetate, and C-PS.[58] Quantitative NMR analysis for O-acetyl content and C-PS of pneumococcal PSs has been examined and

Table 6 Product Release Specifications for Pneumococcal Polysaccharides

Type	Protein (%)	Nucleic Acid (%)	Nitrogen (%)	Phosphorus (%)	O-acetyl (%)	Uronic Acid (%)	Methyl Pentose (%)	Hexosamine (%)	Mol. size CL-4B (%)	CL-2B (%)
1	<2.0	<2.0	3.5-6.0	0-1.5	>1.8	>45	-	-	<0.15	-
2	<2.0	<2.0	0-1.0	0-1.0	-	>15	>38	-	<0.15	-
3	<5.0	<2.0	0-1.0	0-1.0	-	>40	-	-	<0.15	-
4	<3.0	<2.0	4.0-6.0	0-1.5	-	-	-	>40	<0.15	-
5[a]	<7.5	<2.0	3.0-6.0	0-1.5	-	>15	-	>20	-	<0.55
6A(6)	<2.0	<2.0	0-2.0	3.0-4.5	-	-	>15	-	<0.20	-
6B(26)[a]	<2.0	<1.0	0-2.0	2.5-5.0	-	-	>15	-	-	<0.50
7F	<5.0	<2.0	2.0-4.0	0-1.0	-	-	>13	-	<0.20	-
8	<2.0	<2.0	0-1.0	0-1.0	-	>25	-	-	<0.15	-
9N	<2.0	<1.0	2.2-4.0	0-1.0	-	>20	-	>28	<0.20	-
9V(68)[a]	<2.0	<1.0	0.5-3.0	0-1.0	-	>15	-	>14	-	<0.45
10A(34)[a]	<7.0	<1.5	0.8-3.5	1.5-3.5	-	-	-	>12	-	<0.65
11A(43)[a]	<2.0	<1.0	0-2.5	2.0-4.5	>9.0	-	-	-	-	<0.40
12F(12)	<3.0	<2.0	3.0-5.0	0-1.0	-	-	-	>25	<0.25	-
14	<5.0	<2.0	1.5-4.0	0-1.0	-	-	-	>20	<0.25	-
15B(54)[a]	<2.0	<1.0	1.0-3.0	2.0-4.5	-	-	-	>15	-	<0.55
17F(17)[a]	<2.0	<2.0	0-1.5	0-3.5	-	-	-	-	-	<0.45
18C(56)	<3.0	<2.0	0-1.0	2.4-4.9	-	-	>20	-	<0.15	-
19A(57)[a]	<2.0	<2.0	0.6-3.5	3.0-7.0	-	-	>14	>12	<0.45	-
19F	<3.0	<2.0	1.4-3.5	3.0-5.5	-	-	>20	>12.5	<0.20	-
20[a]	<2.0	<1.5	0.5-2.5	1.5-4.0	-	-	>20	>15	-	<0.60
22F(22)[a]	<2.0	<1.0	0-1.0	0-1.0	-	>15	-	-	-	<0.55
23F	<2.0	<2.0	0-1.0	3.0-4.5	-	-	>25	-	<0.15	-
25F(25)	<7.5	<1.0	4.0-5.5	0-2.0	-	-	>37	>31	<0.30	-
33F(70)[a]	<2.5	<1.5	0-2.0	0-1.0	-	-	-	-	-	<0.50

[a]New type.
Data from the Office of Biologics, CBER, Food and Drug Administration, Bethesda, MD.

proposed. Appropriate specifications will be assigned for the tests as the manufacturer obtains more control test data.

A heptavalent conjugate vaccine, Prevnar (licensed to Wyeth–Lederle in 2000), contains seven serotypes (4, 6B, 9V, 14, 18C, 19F, and 23F) individually conjugated to CRM197 protein carrier. The vaccine is adsorbed to aluminum phosphate. Control tests are conducted for various materials used in the manufacturing processes and the final product, including PS, carrier protein, activated saccharide, monovalent conjugate bulk, and 7-valent conjugate final container. These products are analyzed by physicochemical characteristics to ensure their chemical potency, safety, and purity. Testing items and analytical methods for lot release of pneumococcal conjugate vaccine are shown in Table 7.[59]

Nephelometry has been used for quantitation of individual PSs in the pneumococcal PS and conjugate vaccines. This method measures the intensity of scattered light as it passes through the antigen–antibody complex formed by the precipitation reaction. The PS concentration of vaccine samples is determined from the appropriate PS standard curve.

Antibody response data based on serum antibody concentrations in addition to results from an efficacy trial have provided the supporting evidence that an investigational vaccine is associated with protection. Following the recent approval and wide use of Prevnar, conduct of additional efficacy trials in the U.S. has become difficult and would require a very large sample size due to low pneumococcal disease prevalence. In the absence of clinical endpoint efficacy data, it is critical to establish identification of potential immunological correlates of protection and *in vitro* assays to measure these immune parameters. Demonstration of opsonophagocytic activity, avidity to pneumococcal capsular antibody, and antibody duration are important immunologic parameters that could be used as a correlation of protection. Efforts are directed toward developing a standardized assay to assess the opsonophagocytic activity of antipneumococcal antibodies and an ELISA method for antibody quantitation.[60–62] Once standardized and validated analytical methods are developed, direct comparisons of functional activity for different vaccines with corresponding serotype-specific antibody concentrations can be performed.

The next generation of 7- to 11-valent pneumococcal conjugates and their combination vaccines may be approved on the basis of Phase II immunogenicity and safety data. There are possible population-based

Table 7 Control Testing Items and Analytical Methods for Polyvalent Pneumococcal Conjugate Vaccines

Testing Items	Method
I. Polysaccharide (PS)	
Protein	Lowry assay
Nucleic acids	Spectrophotometry
Molecular size	Gel filtration using Sepharose CL-2B and CL-4B or high performance liquid chromatography (HPLC)
C-PS	NMR method
Endotoxin	Limulus amebocyte lysate (LAL) assay
O-acetyl	Colorimetry or NMR method
II. Monovalent conjugate	
Saccharide content	Anthrone assay, nephelometry
Protein content	Lowry assay
Saccharide/protein ratio	
Free saccharide	Separation from bound saccharide and determined by colorimetry
Endotoxin	LAL assay
Molecular size	Gel filtration or HPLC
III. 7-valent conjugate*:	
Saccharide content	Nephelometry
Total saccharide	Anthrone assay
Endotoxin	LAL assay
Sterility	Bacterial culture
General safety	Growth of animals

* 7-valent pneumococcal conjugate vaccine – serotypes 4, 6B, 9V, 14, 18C, 19F, and 23F PSs individually conjugated with CRM197 carrier protein.

From Lee, L.H., Lee, C.J., and Frasch, C.E., Development and evaluation of pneumococcal conjugate vaccines: clinical trials and control tests. *Crit. Rev. Microbiol.*, 28(1):27–41, 2002. With permission.

differences in immune response. This can be evaluated by determining both the quantity and the quality of antibodies after vaccination. A population-based estimate of the level of protective immunity in clinical trials of a 7-valent conjugate vaccine has led to an estimate of a surrogate of protection at an IgG antibody concentration of 0.5 μg/ml serum 1 month after vaccination.[63]

C. Regulatory Actions

After licensure of a drug or biological product, monitoring the safety and effectiveness of the product by the FDA staff continues. Such monitoring and regulatory activity include lot-to-lot release for drugs based on control tests of representative samples of the products performed in FDA's laboratories and review of the manufacturer's test results. Before distribution of a lot of a product to the market, an official release certificate is issued to the manufacturer by the FDA. Furthermore, inspections of many drugs and biological products are conducted annually by FDA scientific and regulatory staff. The purpose of the inspections is to confirm that the products have continued to be manufactured and tested according to the approved license applications, and have followed FDA regulations. Amendments to an approved license application are required for any significant change in the manufacturing procedures, testing, or labeling of the product, as well as changes in manufacturing facilities, equipment, or responsible persons. Such changes must be reported to the FDA 30 days in advance of action. Similarly, major changes in manufacturing methods, test procedures, and labeling require prior approval from the agency before the change can be carried out by the manufacturer.

The FDA may initiate regulatory actions at any time to revoke the manufacturer's license if objectionable conditions and grounds for revocation exist. Such conditions and grounds include the following:

- The licensed product is determined to be no longer safe or effective for its indicated use
- The product or establishment fails to conform to required quality and/or standards
- The establishment or manufacturing process has changed to the extent that the product exerts deleterious effects on public health.
- The manufacturer has failed to report a significant change in facilities, responsible personnel, or in manufacturing procedures and labeling

When the FDA determines that the conditions for license revocation cause an imminent danger or damage to the public health, the agency may immediately suspend a license without notification or hearing. The license may be revoked until the objectionable conditions are resolved. During the period of license suspension, the distribution and sale of the drugs and biological products are prohibited. In many cases, the manufacturer will voluntarily recall the products from the marketplace, when such adverse situations exist. If the recall is considered inadequate, the FDA may take appropriate regulatory action to confiscate the products or issue a court-ordered injunction.

REFERENCES

1. U.S. Government, Elimination of the establishment license application for specified biotechnology and specified synthetic biological products. *Federal Register,* 61, 94, Washington, D.C., U.S. Government Printing Office; 1996:24227–24233.

2. Walsh, G., The drug development process, in *Biopharmaceuticals: Biochemistry and Biotechnology,* John Wiley & Sons, New York, 1998, 37–74.

3. Bugg, C.E., Carson, W.M., and Montgomery, J.A., Drugs by design, *Sci. Am.,* 269(6):92–98, 1993.

4. Biddle, J.A., Technology transfer: what you always wanted to know but were afraid to ask, in *Vaccines — From Concept to Clinic*, Paoletti, L.C. and McInnes, P.M. (Eds.), CRC Press, Boca Raton, FL, 1999, 127–174.

5. The Pharmaceutical Affairs Bureau, Information on the guidelines of toxicity studies required for applications for approval to manufacture (import) drugs. I. *GLP Regulation and Toxicity Tests Guidelines,* Pharmaceutical Affairs Publication Co., Tokyo, 1984, 359.

6. *Code of Federal Regulations*, Nonclinical laboratory studies, good laboratory practice (GLP) regulations, Title 21 part 58, FDA, Rockville, MD, 1991, 233–246.

7. Lee, C.J., Ishimura, K., Nakajima, T., and Huang, J. T., New drug development and good laboratory practice (GLP) in the United States, *Lab. Animal Sci. & Technol.*, 2:95–105, 1990 (Japanese).

8. James, G., FDA's good laboratory practice regulations at home and abroad, presented at Center for Biologics, FDA, Bethesda, MD, October 4, 1988, p. 1–17.

9. Hussein, G. and Bleidt, B., Pharmacokinetics: interactions of new drugs and the human body, in *Clinical Research in Pharmaceutical Development,* Bleidt, B. and Montagne, M. (Eds.), Marcel Dekker, New York, 1997, 109–124.

10. Braeckman, R., Pharmacokinetics and pharmacodynamics of peptide and protein drugs, in *Pharmaceutical Biotechnology,* Crommelin, D.J.A. and Sindelar, R.D. (Eds.), Harwood Academic Publishers, Australia, 1997, 101–120.

11. Baumann, G., Shaw, M.A., and Buchanan, T.A., *In vivo* kinetics of a covalent growth hormone-binding protein complex, *Metabolism,* 38:330–333, 1988.

12. Mohler, M.A., Cook, J.E., and Baumann, G., Binding proteins of protein therapeutics, in *Protein Pharmacokinetics and Metabolism*, Ferraiolo, B.L., Hohler, M.A., and Gloff, C.A. (Eds.), Plenum Press, New York, 1992, 35–71.

13. Chiou, W.L., Ma, C., Chung, S.M. et al., Similarity in the linear and non-linear oral absorption of drugs between human and rat, *Int. J. Clin. Pharm. Ther.,* 38:532–539, 2000.

14. Chiou, W.L. and Barve, A., Linear correlation of the fraction of oral dose absorbed of 64 drugs between human and rats, *Pharm. Res.,* 15:1792–1795, 1998.

15. Chiou, W.L., Jeong, H.Y., Chung, S.M., and Wu, T.C., Evaluation of using dog as an animal model to study the fraction of oral dose absorbed of 43 drugs in humans, *Pharm. Res.*, 17:135–140, 2000.
16. Walter, R.J., Bulk drug substances and purity: a regulatory viewpoint, *Pharm. Technol.*, 10, 35, 1984.
17. Yang, W.H., Statistical treatment of stability data, *Drug Develop. Ind. Pharm.*, 7:63–77, 1981.
18. Center for Drugs and Biologics, Draft guideline for stability studies for human drugs and biologics, 1984. Food and Drug Administration, Rockville, MD, 1984.
19. Grimm, W., Stability testing in industry for world wide marketing, *Drug Develop. Ind. Pharm.*, 12:1259–1292, 1986.
20. Schirmer, R.E., *Modern Methods of Pharmaceutical Analysis,* 2nd ed., CRC Press, Boca Raton, FL, 1991.
21. Adamovids, J.A. (Ed.), *Chromatographic Analysis of Pharmaceuticals*, Marcel Dekker, New York, 1990, 83.
22. Kline, B.J. and Soine, W.H., Gas chromatography: theory, instrumentation, and pharmaceutical applications, in *Pharmaceutical Analysis, Modern Methods*, Munson, J.W. (Ed.), Marcel Dekker, New York. Part A 1981, Part B 1984, 1.
23. Main, K.B. and Medwick, T., Analysis of medicinals, in *Remington's Pharmaceutical Sciences,* 18th ed., Gennaro, A.R. (Ed.), Mark Publishing, Easton, PA, 1990, 435.
24. Flieger, K., Testing in real people, in *New Drug Development in the United States*, Rockville, MD, Food and Drug Administration, 1988.
25. *Code of Federal Regulations*, Investigational new drug application, Title 21, Part 312, Food and Drug Administration, Rockville, MD, 1991, 61.
26. Kessler, D.A., The regulation of investigational drugs, *N. Engl. J. Med.*, 320, 281, 1989.
27. Zivin, J.A., Understanding clinical trials, *Sci. Am.*, 282(4):69–75, 2000.
28. Lo, B., Wolfe, L.E., and Berkeley, A., Conflict-of-interest policies for investigators in clinical trials, *N. Engl. J. Med.*, 343(22):1616–1620, 2000.
29. Martin, J.B. and Kasper D.L., In whose best interest? Breaching the academic-industrial wall, *N. Engl. J. Med.*, 343(22):1646–1649, 2000.
30. Cohn, J.P., The beginnings: laboratory and animal studies, in *New Drug Development in the United States*, Food and Drug Administration, Rockville, MD, 1988, 8–11.
31. www.fda.gov/oc/pdufa/PDUFAIIIgoals.html.
32. *Code of Federal Regulations*, Applications for FDA market approval for a new drug or an antibiotic drug, Title 21, Part 314, Food and Drug Administration, Rockville, MD, 1991, 95–138.
33. Valle, M.A.D., HVAC systems for biopharmaceutical manufacturing plants, *Bio-Pharmacology*, April, 26, 1989.
34. Lee, J.Y., Environmental requirements for clean rooms, *BioPharmacology*, 2, 42, 1989.
35. Bjurstrom, E.E. and Coleman, D., Water systems for biotechnology facilities, *BioPharmacology*, September, 50, 1987.
36. *U.S. Pharmacopoeia*, 23rd ed. Water for pharmaceutical purposes, p. 1984; Sterile water for injection, p. 1636, United States Pharmacopoeial Convention, Rockville, MD, 1995.

37. World Health Organization, Internal drug monitoring: the role of the hospital — a WHO report, *Drug Intell. Clin. Pharm.*, 4:101–110, 1970.
38. *Code of Federal Regulations*, Postmarketing reporting of adverse drug experiences, Title 21, Part 314, Food and Drug Administration, Rockville, MD, 1991, 108–114.
39. Talley, R.B. and Laventurier, M.F., Drug induced illness, *JAMA*, 229:1043, 1974.
40. Stewart, R.B., Adverse drug reactions, in *Remington's Pharmaceutical Sciences*, 18th ed., Gennaro, A.R. (Ed.), Mark Printing Company, Easton, PA, 1990, 1330–1343.
41. Boyer, K.M., Theeravuthichal, J., Vogel, L.C., Orlina, A., and Gotoff, S.P., Antibody response to Group B streptococcus type III and AB blood group antigens, *J. Pediat.*, 98:374–378, 1981.
42. Siber, G.R., Ambrosino, D.M., and Gorgone, G.C., Blood group A-like substances in pneumococcal vaccine, *Ann. Int. Med.*, 96:580–586, 1982.
43. Luzzio, J., Demonstration of blood group substance A bound to *Pasteurella pestis*, *Proc. Soc. Exp. Biol. Med.*, 131:853–858, 1969.
44. Mollison, P.L., Antibodies of the ABO system, in *Blood Transfusion in Clinical Medicine*, 5th ed., Blackwell Scientific Publications, London, 1972, 246–248.
45. Springer, G.F., Blood group A active substances in embrionated chicken eggs and their relation to egg-grown virus, *Science*, 138:687–688, 1962.
46. Springer, G.F., Influenza virus vaccine and blood group A-like substances. Letter to the editor, *Transfusion*, 3:233–236, 1963.
47. Springer, G.F., Shuster, R., and Tritel, H., Influenza vaccine and isoimmunization, *Am. J. Clin. Path.*, 42:589–598, 1964.
48. Oravec, L.S., Lee, C.J., Ann Hoppe, P., and Santos, C.V., Detection of blood group A-like substance in bacterial and viral vaccines by countercurrent immunoelectrophoresis using *Helix pomatia* lectin, *J. Biol Stand.*, 12:159–166, 1984.
49. Faich, G.A., Dreis, M., and Tomita, D., National adverse drug reaction surveillance, 1986, *Arch. Intern. Med.*, 148:785–787, 1988.
50. Rogers, A.S., Israel, E., Smith, C.R., Levine, D., McBean, A.M., Valente, C., and Faich, G., Physician knowledge, attitudes, and behavior related to reporting adverse drug events, *Arch. Intern. Med.*, 148:1595–1600, 1988.
50a. Tanaka, K., Morita, Y., Kawabe, E. et al., Drug use investigation (DUI) and prescription-event monitoring in Japan (J-PEM), *Pharmacoepidemiol. Drug Saf.*, 10(7): 653–658, 2001.
51. Chen, S.T., Re-inventing drug regulation in Asian pacific: the Taiwan experience and a vision for the region, in *Professional Frontiers in the 21st Century*, Lee, C.J. (Ed.), Chinese-American Professionals Association, Washington, D.C., 2002, 3.1–3.5.
52. Chu, M.L., Chern, H.D., Chen, J.J., and Chen, S., Evaluation of drugs and biologics in Taiwan, in *Professional Frontiers in the 21st Century*, Lee, C.J. (Ed.), Chinese-American Professionals Association, Washington, D.C., 2002, 3.6–3.15.
53. Chen, K.C., Building the infrastructure of clinical trials in Taiwan, in *Professional Frontiers in the 21st Century*, Lee, C.J. (Ed.), Chinese-American Professionals Association, Washington, D.C., 2002, 3.16–3.23.
54. Hopps, H.E., Meyers, B.C., and Parkman, P.D., Regulation and testing of vaccines, in *Vaccines*, Plotkin, S.A. and Mortimer, E.A. (Eds.), Saunders Company, Philadelphia, 1988, 576.

55. Adams, W.G. Deaver, K.A., and Cochi, S.L., Decline of childhood *Haemophilus influenzae* type b (Hib) disease in the Hib vaccine era, *JAMA*, 269:221–226, 1993.

56. Lee, C.J., Banks, S.D., and Li, J.P., Virulence, immunity, and vaccine related to *Streptococcus pneumoniae, Crit. Rev. Microbiol.,* 18(2), 89, 1991.

57. World Health Organization, Proposed requirements for pneumococcal polysaccharide vaccine, WHO/BS/79.1251, Rev. 1, Geneva, Switzerland, 1980, 1.

58. Abeygunawardana, C., Williams, T.C., Summer, J.S. et al., Development and validation of an NMR-based identity assay for bacterial polysaccharides, *Anal. Biochem.,* 279:226–240, 2000.

59. Lee, L.H., Lee, C.J., and Frasch, C.E., Development and evaluation of pneumococcal conjugate vaccines: clinical trials and control tests, *Crit. Rev. Microbiol.,* 28(1):27–41, 2002.

60. Lee, C.J., Quality control of polyvalent pneumococcal polysaccharide-protein conjugate vaccine by nephelometry, *J. Biologicals,* 29:1045–56, 2002.

61. Romero-Steiner, S., Libutti, D., Pais, L.B. et al., Standardization of an opsonophagocytic assay for the measurement of functional antibody activity against *Streptococcus pneumoniae* using differentiated HL-60 cells, *Clin. Diag. Lab. Immunol.,* 4:415–422, 1997.

62. Pilikaytis, B.D., Goldblatt, D., Frasch, C.E. et al., An analytical model applied to a multicenter pneumococcal enzyme-linked immunosorbent assay study, *J. Clin. Microbiol.,* 38:2043–2050, 2000.

63. Lee, L.H., Frasch, C.E., Falk, L.A. et al., Correlates of immunity for pneumococcal conjugate vaccines, *Vaccine*, 2003 (in press).

3

PRACTICAL ASPECTS OF DRUG EVALUATION AND RESPONSE

Optimal drug effectiveness and safety is a combination of selecting the appropriate dose and dosing regimen, clear patient instructions, and timely follow-up evaluation. Practical drug therapy depends on continuous drug efficacy and safety monitoring relative to disease status and treatment response. Variable drug response is influenced by internal and external factors. Internal factors consist of considerations such as age, genetic determinants, disease status, physiological conditions of pregnancy, and hormonal balance. External factors include food intake, exposure to environmental chemicals, as well as drug dosage, timing, and route of administration. Hence, in order to choose the appropriate drug, the pharmacokinetic properties of the drug are examined in the context of these internal and external factors.

I. GENERIC AND ORPHAN DRUGS

Most brand-name prescription drugs are developed and manufactured by their innovators, who hold the patents on the drugs. The patent generally lasts about 17 years following the original discovery of the drug. During this time, the company holds an exclusive license from the innovator to sell the drug. Sometimes a drug is so well marketed that it may be better known by the manufacturer's trade name than by its generic name, as in the cases of diazepam (Valium) and furosemide (Lasix). After the patent expires, the right to produce and sell the drug is no longer the exclusive property of the manufacturer who first developed the drug. The drug can then be marketed generically by other companies if they meet certain FDA requirements. These requirements ensure that manufacture of the product's active ingredients continues to be safe and effective.

Drug products are considered to be pharmaceutical equivalents if they contain the same active ingredients and are identical in potency or concentration, dosage form, and route of administration. Products are considered bioequivalent when the bioavailability of the active ingredient in the two products is not significantly different under appropriate test conditions.[1] Bioequivalence is based on equal absorption and biotransformation between a generic and a brand-name drug.

The federal and state governments have enacted legislation to permit and encourage the substitution of a less costly generic equivalent for a more expensive drug during prescription and therapy. The physician, however, can request that a drug not be substituted with its generic equivalent. Generic drug substitution for a pioneer drug product frequently involves two main issues. Is the bioavailability of the generic drug equal to that of its pioneer drug product? Will the patient benefit financially from use of the generic drug?

The Orphan Drug Act defines an orphan drug as a product used for the diagnosis, treatment, or prevention of diseases affecting less than 200,000 people in the U.S. If the prevalence exceeds 200,000 patients in the U.S., the sponsor should show that the cost of development and manufacture of the drug would not be covered by sales from the market. The act was amended several times in 1984, 1985, and 1988. The Office of Orphan Product Development offers grant support for clinical trials of orphan drug research and determines whether submitted requests meet the regulatory requirements for formal review. Written protocol assistance can be obtained from the FDA. Because the incidence of rare diseases is low, correct diagnosis may be delayed. A person could receive ineffective treatment due to misdiagnosed illness. Limited numbers of individuals with rare diseases are available as potential clinical trial participants. Moreover, manufacturers have little incentive to invest in therapeutic drugs, which are costly to develop, for diseases with low incident rates. Sponsors are required to design protocols that permit patient access to therapeutic orphan drugs while the products are still being evaluated in clinical trials.[2]

The act provides various incentives for orphan drug development. These include a tax credit equal to 50% of clinical trial expenses and exclusive marketing rights for 7 years, and have increased the interest in developing orphan drug products.[3,4] Exclusive marketing rights are not the same as a patent. A patent term is 17 years, whereas the duration of exclusive marketing rights is only 7 years. While a product patent covers all product indications, the Orphan Drug Act does not prevent another sponsor from developing the same orphan drug for a different indication. Also, any sponsor can obtain approval of a different orphan drug for the same indication.

Information pertaining to orphan drugs can be obtained from the following sources:

- Within the FDA, the Office of Orphan Product Development provides guidelines to apply for sponsorship of an orphan product or obtain grant support for research on orphan products.
- The National Organization for Rare Disorders provides information about rare diseases, and assists in the start of new support groups and voluntary agencies to help research programs.
- The National Information Center for Orphan Drugs and Rare Diseases provides physicians and pharmacists with orphan drug sponsors' names and telephone numbers.
- The Pharmaceutical Research and Manufacturers of America (PhRMA) provides detailed information about orphan products and sponsors.

Currently, more than 50 FDA-approved orphan drugs are available. Well-recognized products include zidovudine (Retrovir), an antiretroviral drug used to treat persons with HIV; pentamidine (Pentam 300), a prophylactic and therapeutic treatment for *Pneumocystis carinii* pneumonia; and clofazimine (Lamprene), a treatment for resistant leprosy. Orphan drugs and their indications are listed in Table 8.

II. PHARMACOKINETIC MODELS FOR DRUG ABSORPTION

Drug effects are not identical for all individuals. A dose–effect curve applies only to the average of individual responses. A selected drug dose may produce little effect in one person, while producing an excessive effect in another. Population differences are due to variations in rate and extent of drug absorption, distribution, biotransformation, and excretion. The relationship between the toxic and desired effects of a drug is termed a *therapeutic index* (TI). It is usually defined as the ratio of the median toxic dose to the median effective dose, TD50/ED50. In laboratory tests, TI is expressed as the ratio of the median lethal dose over the median effective dose (LD50/ED50). When the TI is large (greater than 3), the variation due to bioavailability is

Table 8   Designated Orphan Products, 1982–1990

Drug/Biologic Name	FDA Sponsor	Approval	Prevalence	Treatment/ Indication
AIDS and Related Diseases				
Ganciclovir sodium (Cytovene)	Syntex	1989	20,000	Cytomegalovirus retinitis in AIDS
Pentamidine isethionate (Pentam 300)	Lyphomed	1984	3,000	*Pneumocystis carinii* pneumonia
(Nebupent)	Lyphomed	1987	17,000	Prevention of *Pneumocystis carinii* pneumonia
Zidovudine (Retrovir)	Burroughs Wellcome	1987	10,000	Treatment of AIDS
			100,000	AIDS-related complex
Cancer				
Etidronate disodium (Didronel)	Norwich Eaton	1987	71,000	Hypercalcemia of malignancy
Ifosfamide (Ifex)	Bristol-Meyers	1988	10,000	Testicular cancer
Interferon-α2a (Roferon-A)	Hoffmann-LaRoche	1988	10,000	AIDS-related Kaposi's sarcoma
Interferon-α2b (Intron A)	Schering	1988	10,000	AIDS-related Kaposi's sarcoma
Mitoxantrone HCl Novantrone)	Lederle Labs	1987	30,000	Acute myelogenous (and non-lymphocytic leukemia
Genetic Diseases				
Alpha-1-proteinase Inhibitor	Cutter Labs	1987	30,000	Congenital inhibitor deficiency
Antithrombin III human (Antithrombin)	Kabi Vitrum	1989	2,500	Hereditary deficiency
L-carnitine (Vitacarn)	Kendall	1986	100	Hereditary deficiency

From Lee, C.J., *Managing Biotechnology in Drug Development*, CRC Press, Boca Raton, 1996. With permission.

not clinically significant. Bioavailability is defined as the rate and extent to which a drug reaches its site of action. For example, suppose the LD50 is very large and the ED50 is very small for a particular drug. This means that the drug has a large LD50/ED50, i.e., only a small dose of a drug is needed to achieve a therapeutic effect in 50% of the population, while a large dose is needed to cause a lethal effect. Thus, from a clinical standpoint, a large variability in absorption will rarely be a concern for the drug to cause a serious toxic effect. On the other hand, when the TI is small, nearly the same dose of drug needed to achieve a therapeutic effect can also cause a lethal effect. Clinically, the physician cannot ignore the variation in bioavailability because even a small variation in drug absorption could induce serious toxicity. The serum levels of drugs such as digitalis, which has a small TI, must thus be monitored very carefully.

A. Bioavailability

In general, the physicochemical properties of the drug, such as solubility, molecular size, and degree of ionization, can influence absorption, all of which affect drug transit across cell membranes. The extent of absorption for a new drug is determined by comparing the area under a drug concentration-time curve (AUC), time to maximum effect (Tmax), and maximum concentration attained (Cmax) relative to reference drug values.

Most drugs are administered orally. They are absorbed from the gastrointestinal tract into the blood and produce a pharmacological effect. The oral route is the most convenient, economical, and safest way to administer drugs. Disadvantages to oral ingestion, however, include the incapability to absorb some drugs due to irritation of the gastrointestinal mucosa, and destruction of drugs by digestive enzymes or low gastric pH. Drugs absorbed through the gastrointestinal tract can be metabolized by mucosal, intestinal, or liver enzymes before reaching the blood circulation (the first-pass effect). The nonionized form of a drug will be absorbed more rapidly than the ionized form at any particular site in the gastrointestinal tract. The intravenous route is advantageous in that the administered dose reaches the blood immediately and becomes completely available. This route also provides an alternative method of delivery for drugs causing severe adverse reactions when given subcutaneously, intramuscularly, or orally. Drugs diluted in solution and distributed in a large blood volume are better tolerated by the body. Blood vessel walls are relatively insensitive to adverse drug effects.

Absorption from subcutaneous and intramuscular injections occurs by simple diffusion along the gradient from drug site to serum. The rate is limited by the area of the absorbing blood capillary and by the drug solubility in the interstitial fluid. The rate of absorption following subcutaneous injection is often constant and slow to provide a sustained effect. The rate of absorption of a suspension, e.g., insulin, is slow compared with that of a soluble preparation of the hormone. Following intramuscular injection, a drug in aqueous solution is absorbed rapidly, and depends on the rate of blood flow to the site. Penicillin is effectively administered in this manner.

Prolonged or controlled-release preparations are formulated to release a drug slowly for 8 hours or longer and thereby increase its duration of action. These dosage forms reduce the frequency of administration of the drug, as compared with conventional dosage forms, and minimize fluctuations in serum drug concentration. Most prolonged-release products are given by oral administration. Drugs that are metabolized through the liver, however, are not suitable to be given orally due to a significant metabolism. Prolonged-release products are produced by several methods, including ion-exchange resins that bind the drug, semipermeable membranes with small laser-drilled holes, slowly eroding coatings or matrices, and slowly dissolving physical or chemical forms.[5]

The rate of drug distribution to tissues is affected by the diffusion rate, tissue perfusion rate, and the extent of plasma and tissue protein binding. The degree of protein binding to albumin is particularly important for acidic drugs, and to α1-acid glycoprotein for basic drugs. Plasma protein binding is a reversible process. The drug molecules constantly shift between the drug–protein complex and the free form, while remaining in overall equilibrium. Although the total amount of drug in plasma changes constantly, the ratio of bound to free drug form remains the same.

The binding of drugs to plasma proteins is nonselective. Hence, interference among drugs with similar physicochemical properties can occur because these drugs compete with each other for the same binding sites. Endogenous substances can compete for these same binding sites as well. For example, the sulfonamides and other organic anions, which are highly bound to plasma proteins, can displace bilirubin from albumin, and thus increase the risk of bilirubin encephalopathy in the newborn. In many cases, the drug toxicity is attributed to competition between drugs for cell binding sites. These drug–drug interactions may also alter elimination of the drug. Competition of drugs for plasma protein-binding sites can also falsely estimate plasma drug concentration, because most assays do not distinguish free drug from the bound form. Lastly, rapid administration of a highly lipid-soluble drug by intravenous or aerosol routes can redistribute a drug from its site of action to other tissues.

Drugs that cross the placenta by simple diffusion can cause congenital defects. Thus, lipophilic nonionized drugs readily enter the fetal blood system from the maternal circulation. A fetus is exposed to essentially all drugs taken by a pregnant mother.

Drug molecules that are more polar and lipid soluble rapidly cross cell membranes during absorption, are more widely distributed, and are consequently excreted in smaller amounts. In contrast, the enzymatic biotransformation of drugs from more polar to less lipid-soluble metabolites enhances their excretion and decreases their volume of distribution. Such biotransformation prevents excessive accumulation of drugs and thereby lessens the chances of drug toxicity.[6,7]

Enzyme systems involved in the biotransformation of drugs are localized in the endoplasmic reticulum of the liver. Chemical reactions of these enzymes are classified as Phase I or Phase II reactions. A Phase I reaction changes the parent drug to a more polar metabolite by oxidation, reduction, or hydrolysis. When the metabolite is converted to a more active drug, the parent compound is called a prodrug; for example, proinsulin is converted to insulin. A Phase II reaction, also known as conjugation, involves the coupling of a drug or its polar metabolite with an endogenous substrate, such as glucuronate, sulfate, acetate, or an amino acid. Drug biotransformation frequently occurs as sequential Phase I and II reactions in the liver and other tissues. A parent drug is converted to several metabolites via consecutive Phase I reaction and Phase II conjugation processes. Drug action is thus prolonged through conversion of the parent compound to an active metabolite. Drug action can be curtailed via conversion to an inactive metabolite, thereby reducing the likelihood of drug toxicity.

Hepatic biotransformation enzymes in the neonate are present in small amounts, particularly in premature babies, because protein synthesis of hepatic enzyme is not fully developed yet. Neonates consequently have reduced ability to conjugate bilirubin, which can result in hyperbilirubinemia and increase the risk to develop encephalopathy. Reduced enzyme activity also increases the toxicity of chloramphenicol and codeine in neonates. An immature blood–brain barrier and excretory system make the fetus and neonate very susceptible to adverse drug effects.

Drugs are removed from the body either unchanged or as metabolites. The body eliminates polar drugs more efficiently than lipophilic compounds. Thus, lipid-soluble drugs are not readily eliminated until they are metabolized to polar compounds. Renal excretion of drugs involves three steps: glomerular filtration, active tubular secretion, and passive tubular reabsorption. The glomerular filtration rate is approximately 125 ml/minute for the average adult. Blood cells and proteins remain in the blood and are not filtered into the renal tubular lumen. Drugs not bound to blood cells and proteins are cleared by glomerular filtration. The maximum rate of drug clearance is equal to the product of the glomerular filtration rate and the fraction of drug unbound in the blood.

The rate of tubular reabsorption depends on the physicochemical properties of the drug. Nonionic lipophilic drugs are extensively reabsorbed. Low urine pH increases renal elimination and is useful in treating overdoses of alkaline drugs. Renal elimination is related to the fraction of drug removed by the kidneys per unit of time. It is affected by kidney function and fraction of unchanged drug excreted into the urine. Changes in kidney function are measured by monitoring endogenous creatinine clearance.[8,9]

B. Pharmacokinetic Models and Their Clinical Applications

Pharmacokinetic properties reflect the ability of a drug to reach a target organ via any route of administration. Organ-specific effect may be dose-dependent.[10,11] Pharmacological activity resulting from the drug's concentration in blood as tissue represents clinical drug effect. In contrast, a toxic response is an observed effect that relates to development of an adverse reaction. Pharmacokinetic models establish a quantitative relationship between dose and effect by measuring drug concentration in biological fluids. Dosing regimens and drug effect are optimized through modification of pharmacokinetic properties.

1. First-Order Elimination

Drug elimination generally proceeds by first-order kinetics; the rate of elimination is proportional to the drug concentration in the body. This process is expressed in the following equation:

$$C = C_0 \cdot e^{-kt} \qquad \text{(Eq. 1)}$$

where k = elimination rate, the slope of the line
C = drug concentration in plasma at any time (t) after its administration
C_0 = initial drug concentration

The drug concentration in plasma can be calculated from this equation. To avoid calculations with exponential components (e), the drug half-life ($t_{1/2}$) is usually used. The half-life is defined as the time required for the drug concentration in serum or plasma to decline by 50%. It is expressed by the following equation:

$$t_{1/2} = 0.693/k \qquad \text{(Eq. 2)}$$

Since half-life changes as a function of both clearance and volume of distribution, Equation 2 may also be expressed as:

$$t_{1/2} = 0.693 \times V/CL \qquad \text{(Eq. 3)}$$

where V = volume of distribution and CL = clearance = (rate of elimination)/C. Clearance of a drug is the ratio of the rate of elimination by all routes to the concentration of drug in certain biological fluids. Creatinine clearance is defined as the rate of elimination of urine creatinine relative to its plasma concentration.

2. Nonlinear Elimination

Sometimes the rate at which drug concentration increases exceeds the maximal capacity of the body to metabolize and/or eliminate the drug; more specifically, a constant amount of the drug is eliminated per unit of time, regardless of the concentration in the body. This process is described as nonlinear elimination. Consequently, increased dosage results in disproportionate increases in plasma drug concentration and in the time required for drug elimination. Modified dose and dosing regimens for propranolol, alcohol, and theophylline are optimally determined by monitoring clinical response. Nonlinear pharmacokinetic properties may be characteristic of drugs that bind to saturable sites in tissues or plasma proteins, or are involved in hepatic metabolism or in active renal transport.

In a practical sense, a drug is usually assumed to be greater than 90% eliminated in about four half-lives. If a drug is administered repeatedly at fixed intervals, accumulation occurs until a plateau is reached. This steady-state concentration, Css, is reached in about four half-lives. Therefore, the longer the half-life of a drug, the longer it will take to reach a plateau level.

The amount of the drug that reaches the blood circulation is expressed as a fraction of the dose F, which is defined as bioavailability. If a drug is metabolized in the liver or excreted in bile, some of the active drug absorbed from the gastrointestinal tract will be inactivated by the liver before it can reach the blood circulation to be distributed to its target sites. The maximum oral availability (Fmax) can be estimated from the following equation:

$$\text{Fmax} = 1 - E = 1 - (\text{CL hepatic}/\text{Q hepatic}) \qquad \text{(Eq. 4)}$$

where E = extraction ratio for a drug across the liver and Q = blood flow.

Therefore, if the hepatic blood clearance for a drug is large relative to hepatic blood flow, the extent of bioavailability will be low when the drug is given orally.

If the values for clearance and bioavailability are measured, the selected dosage for a drug that produces its average steady-state serum concentration can be calculated from the following equation:

$$\text{Dose} = \text{Css} \times \text{CL} \times \tau/F \qquad \text{(Eq. 5)}$$

where CL = clearance, F = bioavailability, and τ = dosing interval. Equation 5 indicates that if clearance is altered in patients with renal or hepatic dysfunction, e.g., very young or old individuals, the dose for a drug should be modified.

If a therapeutic concentration must be achieved rapidly before a period of four half-lives occurs, a loading dose (LD) is required. The loading dose is calculated by the following equation:

$$\text{LD} = C \times Vd/F \qquad \text{(Eq. 6)}$$

where C is a desired serum concentration. There are some disadvantages of using a loading dose: (1) the patient is exposed rapidly to a high concentration of a drug; (2) it will take a long time for the drug concentration to fall when an excessive drug level has been achieved; and (3) large loading doses are often administered rapidly through injection and may induce toxic effects.

C. Regulatory Aspects of Bioequivalence[12,13]

Following extensive efforts of industry, academia, and regulatory agencies, rapid progress has been achieved in development and regulatory evaluation of drug products. Adequate approaches have been established to measure bioavailability and bioequivalence. These approaches ensure product quality over time for both innovative and generic drugs.

Bioequivalence studies assess the relative bioavailability between two products with emphasis on comparative pharmacological activity under similar conditions. Bioequivalence is defined as the absence of significant differences in the rate and extent that an active pharmaceutical ingredient becomes available at the target site. Participants in a bioequivalence study receive test and reference drugs, under fasting conditions, with random assignment to the two possible sequences of administration. Plasma samples are analyzed for concentrations of the drug, and sometimes active metabolites, over a selected time period.

The rate and extent of drug absorption are used to characterize bioequivalence. The U.S. FDA, however, recently recommended a change in the methodology used to assess bioequivalence. Systemic exposure, rather than drug absorption characteristics, is used because absorption measurements are variable, fluctuate over time, and have little clinical relevance. Systemic exposure measurements provide a more comprehensive and consistent absorption profile, which provides greater assurance of therapeutic effect. Systemic exposure measures include total exposure (the area under a drug concentration-time curve, AUC), maximum concentration attained (Cmax), and early exposure (partial AUC from time zero to the peak time of the reference formulation). For some immediate-release drugs, careful assessment of early exposure is important.[14,15]

For drugs in which systemic exposure does not directly relate to safety and efficacy, other approaches, such as comparative pharmacodynamic studies or clinical trials, can be used for assessing bioequivalence. Under certain circumstances, *in vitro* studies can be used to demonstrate bioequivalence. For example, dissolution studies are adequate to demonstrate bioequivalence for highly soluble and permeable drug ingredients formulated in a rapidly dissolving drug product.[16] *In vitro* dissolution test results can also substitute for conventional bioequivalence measures when an *in vitro–in vivo* correlation has been established, or when the requirement for *in vivo* studies is waived for different strengths of a drug product.[17]

Comparison of confidence limits is currently the standard method for determining bioequivalence. Conclusions about bioequivalence have been based on differences between average values.[18] FDA now accepts two additional approaches, population and individual bioequivalence, to support bioequivalence claims.[19,20] These two approaches compare average values and variance. The population bioequivalence method assesses total variance between test and reference products, while individual bioequivalence reflects intra-subject variance and subject-by-formulation interaction.[21] These approaches can be used to analyze both *in vitro* and *in vivo* study results.

III. FACTORS AFFECTING DRUG RESPONSE

The extent of drug response relates to the pharmacological activity of the drug and its metabolites, concentration of active substance at the target site, and the duration for which therapeutic concentrations are maintained. The absorption and bioavailability of a candidate drug is generally assessed in a controlled clinical trial. Although comparative clinical trial conditions are designed to reduce biased interpretation of results, oral drugs given under routine conditions are not so stringent. In many cases, more than one drug is given simultaneously, especially to hospitalized, elderly, or chronically ill individuals. Concomitant drug administration may influence the absorption and clinical response of another drug.

Drug interactions affect gastrointestinal absorption and subsequent drug concentration in the blood. Some interactions cause reduced absorption of a given compound. Indirect factors affecting drug absorption include gastric motility, transit time from the stomach to the small intestine, and mucosal integrity of the colon. Any drug that affects gut motility will influence the absorption of other drugs. Propantheline has anticholinergic activity, which reduces gut motility and stomach-emptying rate. Metoclopramide, in contrast, increases the stomach-emptying rate. Both drugs have significant opposing effects on absorption of other medications: (1) metoclopramide increases the absorption rates of acetaminophen, ethanol, and lithium; and (2) propantheline decreases the absorption rate of ethanol, hydrochlorothiazide, and lithium.[22] Some drugs directly affect drug absorption. Antacids increase gastric pH, which increases the solubility of acids and decreases the solubility of bases. Antacids may also adsorb or chelate drugs, forming soluble or insoluble complexes, which in turn affect stomach-emptying rate. Cholestyramine, an anionic exchange resin, binds to cholesterol metabolites and bile acids in the intestinal lumen, prevents their reabsorption, and thus depletes body cholesterol.[23] The interaction between metal ions and oral tetracyclines is well-recognized and clinically relevant. A dramatic reduction in tetracycline serum concentrations occurs in the presence of ferrous sulfate.[24] The degree of interaction depends on the interim time interval following drug administration and the formation of ferrous ion derivatives.

A. External Factors: Diet, Environmental Chemicals, Lifestyle

Humans are exposed daily to a wide range of environmental chemicals. Exposure to environmental factors extrinsically influences drug absorption and biotransformation rates. The choice of dietary intake greatly impacts drug absorption, distribution, metabolism, and elimination. The amount of dietary fat can affect absorption of lipid-soluble drugs. Charcoal-broiled meat, which contains polycyclic hydrocarbons, reportedly causes marked decrease in the bioavailability of phenacetin, but enhances the oxidative biotransformation rates of antipyrine and theophylline. These effects can be avoided by choosing alternative sources of dietary protein and carbohydrate. Severe vitamin and protein deficiencies also affect drug binding and biotransformation.[25] The majority of dietary interactions decreases the rate or extent of drug absorption, which can be beneficial or detrimental.[26] Griseofulvin taken with fatty foods enhances drug absorption. Headache and rebound hypertension occur in individuals taking monoamine oxidase inhibitors who also eat cheese, liver, meats, or beans, all of which contain tyramine. Ingestion of iron preparations or potassium salts with meals reduces gastrointestinal irritation. Dietary supplements, however, unpredictably affect drug metabolism and response.[27] Variable effects of diet on drug interactions necessitate specific instructions (e.g., medications taken before or after a meal) to maximize therapeutic response. Tetracycline, penicillin, cephalosporins, and erythromycin are taken while the stomach is empty to achieve high drug levels in the blood. Chlorothiazide, propranolol and esters of erythromycin are more efficiently absorbed when taken after meals.

Lifestyle choices for cigarette use, alcohol consumption, and foods containing additives are also factors that affect pharmacologic activity of a drug. Cigarettes contain polycyclic hydrocarbons that induce hepatic oxidases, particularly in young people.[28] The increased enzymatic activity and metabolism necessitates the increase in the dosage of theophylline. Cigarette smoking also decreases the urinary excretion of nicotine, lowers plasma levels of phenacetin, theophylline, imipramine, and antipyrine. Other chlorinated hydrocarbons in pesticides, such as DDT, can increase the biotransformation of antipyrine and theophylline.[29] Alcohol has many properties that alter the response to drugs. The interaction between alcohol and drugs is sadly well known. Alcohol use inhibits the biotransformation of many drugs by inducing microsomal oxidation enzymes.[30,31]

B. Intrinsic Factors: Genetic Determinants

Intrinsic factors also affect individual response to drugs. Because genetic determinants vary for each individual, drug response for any given dose may not be uniform. Few drugs are excreted unchanged. Thus, for the majority of drugs, biotransformation rate to an inactive metabolite depends on genetic composition. Biotransformation studies of heterocyclic antidepressants in heterozygous twins showed that the variability in drug response is controlled by genetic determinants.[32] Genetic differences may also alter functional activity of the parent drug. Some drugs are converted via acetylation to either an inactive (e.g., N-acetylisoniazid) or active metabolite (e.g., N-acetylprocainamide). Individuals are categorized as slow or fast acetylators. Rapid acetylators are homozygous or heterozygous for a gene which quickly inactivates an acetylating enzyme, while slow acetylators have a homozygous recessive determinant. About 50% of American whites and blacks are slow inactivators of isoniazid, whereas few Asians and Eskimos have this genetic trait. Liver damage is more frequent in rapid acetylators, perhaps due to the accumulation of a metabolite of isoniazid, acetylhydrazine, which is converted to an acylating agent that induces hepatocellular necrosis in these individuals. Elevated plasma levels of isoniazid in slow acetylators may cause dose-related neuropathies and interfere with the biotransformation of other drugs. Hence, by identifying the acetylator phenotype, therapeutic failure or adverse reactions can be avoided. Drug oxidation appears to be regulated by two alleles at a single gene locus. Persons with glucose-6-phosphate dehydrogenase (G6PD) deficiency have the potential to develop hemolytic anemia if given oxidant drugs. Antimalarial drugs such as primaquine, pamaquine, and pentaquine, sulfonamides, antipyretic medication, chloramphenicol, aminosalicylic acid, and vitamin K oxidize enzyme-deficient red blood cells and hemolysis results. Oxidant drugs usually cause more severe anemia in G6PD-deficient Caucasian individuals than in African-American individuals with the same condition.[32,33] Pharmacogenetic research has made efforts to determine whether a genetic basis for differences in drug response exists, and also to concentrate on developing diagnostic methods to identify susceptible patients.

C. Intrinsic Factors: Age and Disease Conditions

The relative mass of subcutaneous tissue peaks at 9 months of age, declines until about 6 years of age, and then increases again during adolescence. These changes affect the distribution of lipid-soluble drugs. Renal dysfunction can alter the distribution, metabolism, and excretion of drugs. Changes in drug distribution can be classified into two types: (1) effects that change the total plasma concentration of the drug, e.g., warfarin, digoxin, and (2) effects that modify free plasma fraction, e.g., salicylates, phenobarbital. The volume of distribution of digoxin is significantly reduced by severe kidney disease. Impaired drug distribution occurs in individuals with uremia or nephritic syndrome due to changes in urine pH or altered protein binding. Hypoalbuminemia decreases the protein binding of drugs such as warfarin, sulfonamides, and penicillin. As a result, greater amounts of unbound drug are present, which in turn increases the level of circulating active drug. Increased serum levels augment pharmacologic activity, or worse, may cause toxic adverse reactions. Decreased protein binding likewise intensifies the activity of diazoxide and thiopental. Systemic acidosis in uremia patients also causes increases in central nervous system permeability, which further perpetuates potential toxicity to salicylates and phenobarbital.[34,35]

The liver may clear a drug from the body by excreting it in unchanged form into the biliary tract, or as an inactive metabolite that is readily excreted in the urine. Impaired hepatic function likewise impairs drug elimination. Metabolic capacity is reduced by hepatic necrosis. Medications may need to be adjusted for individuals with hepatic dysfunction. Doses for these individuals frequently are decreased for oral medicines, medicines metabolized extensively by the liver, or drugs with a narrow therapeutic index.[36,37]

Age affects drug response. Neonatal renal and hepatic organ systems are normally not completely mature at birth, and organ function naturally wanes in the elderly. The pharmacokinetics of drug absorption and elimination, volume of distribution, and receptor sensitivity in these populations differ from those in healthy adults. Immature hepatic function implies that protein synthesis is not fully functional in infants. Lower concentrations of plasma proteins are associated with decreased plasma protein binding. Salicylates, penicillins, phenobarbital, and sulfonamides compete with bilirubin, which is highly protein bound, for existing binding sites. Consequently, pharmacological activity increases due to increased levels of free (active) drug. Until physiological function and metabolic mechanisms fully develop, dosing regimens for premature infants and neonates should be adjusted to prevent excess accumulation. Infants also have impaired gastric function, greater proportion of body water, and less hepatic metabolic capacity compared to adults. Because the gastric acidity is decreased in newborns, there is increased absorption of acid-labile penicillins. In older children, decreased gastric acidity enhances the rate of absorption of anticonvulsants and imipramine.

Women taking medication during pregnancy may potentially affect maternal health and fetal development. A pregnant woman who receives a drug that increases induction of maternal liver enzymes shortens the plasma half-life of the drug. Fetal kidneys are slow to eliminate drugs that cross the placenta. Thus, drug doses must be carefully adjusted to avoid accumulation and adverse reactions. Pediatric dosing regimens may be calculated based on mg/kg of body weight, mg/M of body surface area (bsa), or as a fraction of an adult dose. General formulas for calculating pediatric drug dose are based on proportions of body weight ($Wt^{0.7}$; Wt (lb) $\times 0.055$). For some drugs, the dosage expressed as mg per square meter of surface area rather than per unit of body weight may provide a more accurate method of adjusting the dose to the age of the patient.[38,39]

Elderly adults consume many more drugs than young adults. Two thirds of Americans older than 65 are taking at least one prescription drug; of those who take prescription drugs, at least one third take three or more.[40] Thus, physicians prescribing medications, particularly for the elderly, are mindful of possible drug interactions. Choice of drug, dose, and dosing regimen are carefully considered.

A gradual deterioration of body systems naturally occurs with age. Absorption of nutrients, vitamins, and minerals is not as active. Supplemental doses of iron, calcium, thiamine, galactose, and vitamin B12 may then be needed.[41] Decreased blood circulation and changes in body composition inevitably affect the distribution and equilibration rate of drugs. Plasma albumin level may also decline, which increases the free fraction of drugs. Hepatic enzyme oxidative capacity declines with age, and such tendency is greater in elderly men than in elderly women.[42]

Kidneys become less functional with increasing age. Decreased renal blood flow results in decreased creatinine clearance. In addition, many patients over 60 years of age have kidney disease, which further reduces renal function. Therefore, it is important to evaluate a person's renal function when selecting the dose of certain drugs; the serum drug concentration should also be monitored carefully. Normal decline in glomerular filtration rate during aging is not reflected by decreases in serum creatinine. A proportional loss in muscle mass also occurs, which decreases creatinine production. Since decreases in glomerular filtration rate and creatinine production are roughly proportional, the serum creatinine level remains unchanged.

IV. MECHANISMS OF DRUG INTERACTION

Mechanisms of drug interaction are multifactorial. A drug interaction is defined as a modified effect of one drug by prior or concomitant administration of another drug. The pharmacological response for a combination of two or more drugs is not always directly proportional to an individual drug's effect. Drug potentiation occurs when the resultant response of these drug combinations is greater than the sum of their separate actions. If the overall result is less than expected, the combination of drugs is antagonistic. Drug effects that are additive or synergistic are clinically important, especially for treatment of antibiotic-resistant organisms, polymicrobial infections, and as an initial choice for febrile neutropenic individuals. Other examples include probenecid, which prolongs the activity and improves the effectiveness of penicillin, and diuretics, which enhance the activity of antihypertensive drugs.

Mechanisms of drug interactions can be divided into those involving (1) chemical or physical incompatibility; (2) pharmacokinetic effect on absorption, distribution, biotransformation, and/or excretion; and (3) pharmacodynamic response, e.g., one drug alters the action of a second drug at the receptor site. Direct physical or chemical inactivation of drugs occurs during exposure of riboflavin or ascorbic acid to light, neutralization of acidic and alkaline drugs mixed in the same container, and during storage conditions resulting in oxidation or elevated temperature. Conditions that affect physical and/or chemical binding in the gastrointestinal tract, slow intestinal motility, or alter gastric pH or enteric flora impact bioavailability. For example, cholestyramine resin adsorbs digoxin and thyroid hormone, thereby reducing absorption of both drugs. Elevation of gastric pH by administering sodium bicarbonate decreases the absorption of tetracycline. Oral neomycin changes the bacterial flora and thereby decreases the absorption rate of simultaneously administered digoxin. Decreased bioavailability reduces the potency and available quantity of active drug.

For most drugs, the plasma concentration of free drug, rather than the total concentration, correlates with the pharmacological activity. Protein-bound drugs can be displaced by other drugs or chemical agents. Changes in the bound fraction temporarily increase the free drug concentration and enhance activity until re-equilibrium is reached. Serious complications can occur when a highly bound drug requiring biotransformation for inactivation is displaced in a patient with hepatic or renal dysfunction. Phenylbutazone, for example, potentiates the anticoagulation activity of warfarin. Phenylbutazone displaces protein-bound warfarin in the plasma, and also inhibits hepatic biotransformation; elevated concentration of free warfarin and delayed hepatic excretion prolong bleeding.[43]

Induction and inhibition of hepatic cytochrome P-450 enzymes and microsomal oxidases are well-known focal points for drug interaction. The rate of metabolite formation, subsequent detoxification, and elimination from the body are affected, as well as oxidation, reduction, hydrolysis, and conjugation processes. Phenobarbital, rifampin, alcohol, and phenylbutazone are all potent cytochrome P-450 enzyme inducers. The therapeutic effect of disulfiram is based on its ability to inhibit the oxidation of acetaldehyde. Allopurinol is a xanthine oxidase inhibitor, an enzyme involved in purine metabolism; serum mercaptopurine concentrations consequently increase.

Kidney function largely influences mechanisms of drug interaction. Aminoglycosides, when coadministered with methoxyflurane, potentiates renal dysfunction. Tubular reabsorption is sensitive to tubular fluid pH; both reabsorption and secretion are affected by competition between drugs and normal metabolites. Anionic metabolites, uric acid, sulfonamides, glucuronide conjugates, and penicillin are all eliminated by the same transport system and thus can competitively block each other's excretion.

A. Receptor Sites of Drug Action

There are many examples of pharmacodynamic interactions in drug therapy. Drug interactions, initiated by membrane-bound receptor, ion channel, and transport site activation, broadly impact important biologic functions. The receptor site is the drug binding site that facilitates recognition and subsequent signal transduction. Receptor site activation sometimes triggers negative feedback mechanisms that reduce the response to a concomitantly administered drug. The muscarinic cholinergic receptor mediates anticholinergic effects of heterocyclic antidepressants, antihistamines, and phenothiazines, all through the same receptor.

Cell-surface proteins, the most important class of drug receptors, are essential components of the main metabolic and regulatory pathways (e.g., dihydrofolate reductase, acetylcholinesterase) that are involved in transport processes (e.g., Na+, K+-ATPase) or structural roles. Receptor binding affinity depends on the type of chemical bond. Most interactions between drugs and receptors involve bonds of multiple types, which include ionic, hydrogen, hydrophobic, van der Waals, and covalent. If binding is covalent, the duration of drug action is frequently prolonged. High affinity, noncovalent binding appears to be essentially irreversible.[44,45]

For small molecules that interact with cell-surface proteins to elicit a therapeutic effect, the conformation of the binding site is crucial. The chemical structure of endogenous agonists was used to map the structure of the receptor binding site, which in turn was used to develop β-adrenergic and histamine H2-receptor antagonists.[46] Cloning, gene sequencing, and site-directed mutagenesis techniques provided the tools to mimic highly specific binding sites. Mutagenic studies on the β-adrenoceptor gene showed that substitution of Asp79 with Asn had no effect on antagonist binding to the human β-adrenergic receptor, but produced a 240-fold loss in affinity of the receptor for norepinephrine.[47] A substitution of Asn at position 130 had no effect on antagonist binding but elicited a tenfold higher affinity for agonists.[48] These studies indicated that agonists and antagonists bind to different sites on the same receptor. It is well known that disease conditions have resultant end-organ effects. Regulation of metabolic function is highly sensitive to stress. Complex feedback mechanisms control the density of hormone and neurotransmitter receptors. There are three locations on the cell surface where physiological and pathological modulation of hormone, neurotransmitter, and drug effects can take place: the receptor, the receptor coupling proteins (GTP-activated proteins), and cell membrane lipid bilayer. The end result of the processed signal from hormones, neurotransmitters, or drug activity is regulated either by concentration of membrane receptors or that of the transduction of G-protein-linked receptors. Maturation effects and pathological processes modify patterns of organ response to hormones, neurotransmitters, and drug interactions. Bacterial components can also directly intervene at the cell surface level. *Vibrio cholera* toxin directly binds to G-protein receptors, persistently activates adenylate cyclase, and ultimately causes life-threatening diarrhea. The pathophysiologic mechanism involves adenosine diphosphate (ADP)-ribosylation of Gs-protein.[49] *Escherichia coli* enterotoxin also acts through the same mechanism to produce diarrhea.[50] Significant loss of Gi-protein expression, however, has also been observed in livers of diabetic rats.[51] Receptor activation and modulation hence are highly cell-specific and complicate interpretation of observed drug actions.[52]

B. Structure–Activity Relationship of Drugs

Receptor binding affinity and intrinsic drug action are closely related to a drug's molecular structure. Subtle changes in stereoisomerism, or side chains, can affect pharmacological activity. Greater understanding of structure–activity relationships have led to the synthesis and production of valuable therapeutic agents. Changes in molecular configuration do not affect all drug actions equally, thus, it is possible to develop a new compound with a more favorable ratio of therapeutic to toxic effects, enhanced specificity to tissues, or more stable characteristics than those of the parent drug. Many effective hormone and neurotransmitter antagonists have been developed by this method. Minor modifications of structure also induce profound effects on the pharmacokinetic properties of drugs.

The most frequent therapeutic approach in drug development is to synthesize analogs of known effective drugs. Specific pharmacological activity depends on properties of more than one functional group. Ideal properties needed for optimal action at the receptor include drug molecule size, shape, degree of ionization, and orientation of charged groups. Parameters for synthetic analogs are carefully duplicated using computational chemistry, quantitation of structure–activity relationships, and molecular modification of a parent molecule. Structure–activity relationship studies help to determine the molecular site of pharmacological activity and also to develop drugs with increased potency, greater selectivity, prolonged duration of action, and lower toxicity.[5,53]

V. ADVERSE DRUG REACTIONS

Adverse drug reactions are classified as expected local and system reactions, unpredictable idiopathic responses, or immediate hypersensitivity reactions. These reactions are temporally, but not always causally, related to drug ingestion. Expected adverse reactions are exaggerated pharmacological outcomes when a drug is given in therapeutic doses. Hypoglycemia is a known complication of antidiabetic drugs, hypotension with antihypertensive agents, and hemorrhage with anticoagulants. Idiopathic reactions involve unanticipated aberrant effects from the described profile of pharmacological actions at therapeutic drug doses; the mechanism leading to the adverse outcome is not known. Glucocorticoid glaucoma, chloramphenicol-induced aplastic anemia, malignant hyperthermia associated with anesthesia, and immunologic hypersensitivity are all examples of this type of adverse reaction. Hypersensitivity reactions have causes that include (a) decomposition of the active component; (b) effects of additives, solubilizers, or stabilizers incorporated in drug preparations; and (c) effects from by-products of the active constituents. Although information about local and systemic adverse reactions is well characterized, rare acute and long-term events usually are identified through postmarketing surveillance. Prelicensure trials assess drug safety in approximately 1000 to 3000 subjects. The probability of identifying an adverse drug reaction with a frequency of less than 1:1000 is therefore extremely low. Under conditions of widespread, routine and long-term use, less frequent events can be detected.

A. Causal Relationship between Drugs and Adverse Reactions

Most drugs have more than one pharmacological action, some of which may be responsible for both desired therapeutic effects and adverse reactions. Whether the effect produced is desired or undesired, the underlying pharmacologic mechanism responsible for the outcome may be the same. For example, the dose of digoxin needed to induce a desirable therapeutic effect on the cardiovascular system may also produce a toxic effect on the gastrointestinal system.[53,54] Adverse drug reactions are often induced by drug hypersensitivity. Allergic reactions to drugs result from specific antibodies and delayed cellular hypersensitivity, which releases histamine or other chemical mediators responsible for tissue injury. Multiple factors predispose an individual to adverse drug effects. These factors include the dose, the inherent toxicity of the agent, age, gender, genetic composition, drug compliance, disease status, and concomitantly administered medications. Drug dose and pharmacokinetic properties are major toxicologic determinants. Elderly people often suffer much higher incidences of adverse reactions because they take a greater number and greater variety of medications, and often suffer from a reduced general health status. Approximately 50% of the deaths reported to the FDA as adverse reactions occurred in patients 60 years and older.[55] Ethnic background and genetic susceptibility to the toxic effects of succinylcholine, isoniazid, and monoamine oxidase inhibitors were minor factors.[56] Multiple-drug therapy is also a prominent factor leading to prolonged complications in hospitalized patients. For example, the average number of drugs given to hospitalized patients is 8.4.[57] Patients who undergo frequent diagnostic testing can also develop adverse reactions to adjunct medication. Thus, decreasing exposure to an increased number of drugs is a simple method to reduce adverse reactions.

Defined criteria have been established by the FDA's Division of Epidemiology and Surveillance to assess possible causal relationships between adverse reactions and drug administration.[58,59] These criteria involve the following questions: (1) Did the adverse reaction of a suspected drug follow a reasonable temporal sequence? (2) Did the patient improve after removal of the drug? (3) Did the adverse reaction appear when administration of the drug was resumed? (4) Could the reaction be reasonably explained by the known characteristics of the patient's clinical state? Based on the responses, causality of the adverse reaction is classified as follows:

- *Highly probable*: a reaction that follows a reasonable temporal sequence after administration of the drug; that follows a known response pattern when the dose of the drug is reduced (dechallenge) and reappearance of the reaction on repeated exposure (rechallenge); that the reaction can be explained by known characteristics of a person's clinical state
- *Probable*: a reaction that follows a reasonable temporal sequence after administration of the drug; that follows a known response pattern to the suspected drug (confirmed by dechallenge), but could not be explained by the known characteristics of the person's clinical state
- *Possible*: a reaction that follows a reasonable temporal sequence after administration of the drug and follows a known response pattern to the suspected drug; but that could have been produced by the person's clinical state or other modes of given therapy
- *Not related*: any reaction that does not meet the criteria above, especially if the event has no reasonable temporal association with use of the drug

Adverse reactions may be prevented as follows:[54,60]

- Optimize drug therapy by giving the necessary, least number of drugs that achieve the desired effect. Do not use drugs in a pregnant patient unless the drug benefit outweighs the risk of adverse reaction.
- Instruct patients to identify early signs and symptoms associated with adverse reactions and to contact the physician immediately when these symptoms are found. Ask if the patient has had previous reactions.

- Ask if the patient is self-medicating with herbal supplements. Avoid deleterious drug interactions.
- Consider giving smaller doses to subpopulations of elderly, infants, and those with hepatic or renal impairment.
- Repeat directions to the elderly and others likely to misunderstand dosing instructions. Use a familiar drug.

B. Adverse Reaction during Pregnancy and Lactation

Recently, it has been realized that many drugs administered to a mother during pregnancy and lactation may adversely affect the fetus and infant. A neonate is less capable than an adult to biotransform and excrete drugs, and is thus more susceptible to an adverse reaction.

The placenta is a metabolically active tissue that contains enzymes involved in the active transport of substances across membranes, intermediary metabolism, and biotransformation of drugs. The placental barrier is a relative one, and any drug present in overwhelming concentration in the maternal circulation will be transferred to the fetus.[61] The mechanism involved in the placental transfer of drugs is mainly simple diffusion. The rate of diffusion is controlled by the concentration gradient of the drug, diffusion constant of the agent, the surface area available for transfer, and the thickness of the placental membrane. Drugs with low molecular weights (less than 600) cross the placenta relatively easily. Drugs that are un-ionized and highly lipid soluble diffuse more rapidly than those that are highly ionized and less lipid soluble. Besides simple diffusion, other mechanisms of membrane transfer, such as facilitated diffusion and active transport, may also be involved in the passage of drug across the placenta.

The first trimester of gestation is the stage that organogenesis occurs in the embryo. Drugs administered during this crucial developmental period are highly likely to cause congenital malformations (teratogenic effect). If the malformation is lethal, abortion usually results. The most critical period for causing gross congenital defects is when the gestational age of the fetus is between 21 and 31 days.[62] Other contributory factors include the drug's chemical properties, its accessibility in unbound form, the dose and duration of action, interactions of concomitantly administered drugs, and genetic and environmental determinants.[63] Teratogenic effects in humans were identified by a unique pattern of birth defects caused by drugs such as thalidomide, warfarin, penicillamine, and diethylstilbestrol. Many mechanisms of teratogenesis are not fully understood. At present, it is rarely possible to predict teratogenicity on a pharmacological basis. Toxic drug effects cause congenital malformations directly (e.g., thalidomide); indirectly, by inhibition of metabolism (by folic acid antagonists) or through hormone imbalance (by estrogens); by effecting maternal nutrition or health status (by psychotropic drugs); and by effecting the fetoplacental system (e.g., cortisone may induce cleft palate by reducing amniotic fluid volume, resulting in bending of the head so that the tongue prevents palatal closure).[64] Five categories were established to inform the general public of prescription drug risk during pregnancy.[65] Drugs known to have a potential harm to the fetus are divided into the following risk levels:

- **Pregnancy category A.** Controlled studies in women fail to demonstrate a risk to the fetus in the first trimester, and the possibility of fetal harm appears remote.
- **Pregnancy category B.** Animal reproduction studies have not demonstrated a fetal risk but there are no controlled studies in pregnant women, or animal reproduction studies have shown an adverse effect that was not confirmed in controlled studies in women in the first trimester.
- **Pregnancy category C.** Animal studies have revealed adverse effects on the fetus and there are no controlled studies in women, or studies in women and animals are not available. Drugs in this category should be given only if the potential benefit justifies the risk to the fetus.
- **Pregnancy category D.** There is positive evidence of human fetal risk, but the benefits for pregnant women may be acceptable despite the risk, as in life-threatening or serious diseases for which safer drugs cannot be used or are ineffective.
- **Pregnancy category X.** Studies in animals or humans have demonstrated fetal abnormalities, there is evidence of fetal risk based on human experience, or both, and the risk of using the drug in pregnant women clearly outweighs any possible benefit. The drug is contraindicated in women who are or may become pregnant.

Drugs administered during the second and third trimesters of pregnancy are unlikely to be teratogenic, since organogenesis is already complete. Instead, drugs affect organ growth and function. Drugs given late in pregnancy likewise may be lethal to a fetus. Usually, the fetus is more sensitive to the toxic effects of drugs than the mother. However, in life-threatening conditions affecting the mother, the treatment of maternal disease should be weighed against adverse effects on the fetus. Neonates, particularly if born prematurely, are very susceptible to adverse drug reactions. For example, the toxic effects of chloramphenicol in neonates are caused by deficient metabolism, delayed renal excretion, and increased cell penetration. In addition, a neonate may be affected by drugs taken by the mother during lactation. Almost all drugs present in the maternal circulation are transferred to breast milk; the maximum amount of drug, however, secreted into milk is usually less than 2% of the maternal dose. Maternal use of cyclosporine and radioactive drugs is contraindicated during breast-feeding. Lithium is considered to be contraindicated; sulfonamides, antithyroid drugs, and iodides are relatively contraindicated.[66–68]

REFERENCES

1. *Code of Federal Regulations*, Bioequivalence requirements, Title 21, Part 320, Food and Drug Administration, Rockville, MD, 1991, 151–157.
2. Haffner, M.E., Orphan products: origins, progress, and prospect, *Annu. Rev. Pharmacol. Toxicol.*, 31, 603, 1991.
3. Cato, A.E., Stang, P., and Sutton, R.O., Orphan drug development: David and Goliath, in *Clinical Drug Trials and Tribulations*, Cato, A.E. (Ed.), Marcel Dekker, New York, 1988, 227.
4. Orphan drugs, in *Drug Evaluations Annual 1991*, American Medical Association, Milwaukee, WI, 1991, 67.
5. Gibalde, M., Prolonged-release medication, *Perspect. Clin. Pharmacol.*, 2:17–53, 1984.
6. Goldstein, A., Aronow, L., and Kalman, S.M., *Principles of Drug Action: The Basis of Pharmacology*, 2nd ed., John Wiley & Sons, New York, 1974.
7. Jacquz, E., Hall, S.D., and Branch, R.A., Genetically determined polymorphisms in drug oxidation, *Hepatology*, 6:1020–1032, 1986.
8. Anders, M.W., Metabolism of drugs by the kidney, *Kidney Int.*, 18:636–647, 1980.
9. Cockcroft, D.W. and Gault M.H., Prediction of creatinine clearance from serum creatinine, *Nephron*, 16:31–41, 1976.
10. Rowland, M. and Tozer, T.N., *Clinical Pharmacokinetics: Concepts and Applications*, 2nd ed., Lea & Febiger, Philadelphia, 1989.
11. Matzke, G.R. and St. Peter, W.L., Clinical pharmacokinetics 1990, *Clin. Pharmacokinet.*, 18 (1):1–19, 1990.
12. Chen, M.L., Regulatory overview of bioavailability and bioequivalence, in *Professional Frontiers in the 21st Century*, Lee, C.J. (Ed.), Chinese-American Professionals Association, Washington, D.C., 2002, 3.43–3.47.
13. Malinowski, H.J., Bioavailability and bioequivalence testing, in *Remington: The Science and Practice of Pharmacy*, 20th ed., Gennaro, A.R. (Ed.), Lippincott Williams & Wilkins, Baltimore, MD, 2000, 995–1004.

14. U.S. Food and Drug Administration, Center for Drug Evaluation and Research. *Guidance for Industry: Bioavailability and Bioequivalence Studies for Orally Administered Drug Products – General Considerations*, Office of Training and Communications, Division of Communications Management, Drug Information Branch, HFD-210, Rockville, MD, October 2000.

15. Chen, M.L., Lesko, L.J., and Williams, R.L., Measure of exposure versus measures of rate and extent of absorption, *Clin. Pharmacokinet.*, 40(8):565–572, 2001.

16. U.S. Food and Drug Administration, Center for Drug Evaluation and Research. *Guidance for Industry: Waiver of In Vivo Bioavailability and Bioequivalence Studies for Immediate Release Solid Oral Dosage Forms Based on a Biopharmaceutics Classification System*, Office of Training and Communications Management, Drug Information Branch, HFD-210, Rockville, MD, August 2000.

17. U.S. Food and Drug Administration, Center for Drug Evaluation and Research. *Guidance for Industry: Extended Release Oral Dosage Forms: Development, Evaluation, and Application of In Vitro/In Vivo Correlation*, Office of Training and Communications, Division of Communications Management, Drug Information Branch, HFD-210, Rockville, MD, September 1997.

18. Schuirmann, D.J., A comparison of the two one-sided tests procedure and the power approach for assessing the bioequivalence of average bioavailability, *J. Pharmacokinet. Biopharm.*, 15:657–680, 1987.

19. U.S. Food and Drug Administration, Center for Drug Evaluation and Research. *Guidance for Industry: Statistical Approaches to Establishing Bioequivalence*, Office of Training and Communications, Division of Communications Management, Drug Information Branch, HFD-210, Rockville, MD, January 2001.

20. Chen, M.L., Patnaik, R., Hauck, W.W. et al., An individual bioequivalence criterion: regulatory considerations, *Stat. Med.*, 19:2821–2842, 2000.

21. Hauck, W.W., Hyslop, T., Chen, M.L. et al., Subject-by-formulation interaction in bioequivalence: conceptual and statistical issues, *Pharm. Res.*, 17:375–380, 2000.

22. Welling, P.G., Interactions affecting drug absorption, *Clin. Pharmacokinet.*, 9:404–434, 1984.

23. Moore, R.B., Crane, C.A., and Frantz, Jr., I.D., Effect of cholestyramine on the fecal excretion of intravenously administered cholesterol-4-14C and its degradation productions in a hypercholesterolemic patient, *J. Clin. Invest.*, 47:1664–1671, 1968.

24. Neuvonen, P.J. and Turakka, H., Inhibitory effect of various iron salts on the absorption of tetracycline in man, *Eur. J. Clin. Pharm.*, 7:357–360, 1974.

25. Alvares, A.P., Pantuck, E.J., Anderson, K.E., Kappas, A., and Conney, A.H., Regulation of drug metabolism in man by environmental factors, *Drug Metab. Rev.*, 9(2):185–205, 1979.

26. Welling, P.G., Interactions affecting drug absorption, *Clin. Pharmacokinet.*, 9:404–434, 1984.

27. Campbell, T.C. and Hayes, J.R., Role of nutrition in the drug-metabolizing enzyme system, *Pharmacol. Rev.*, 26:171–197, 1974.

28. Vestal, R.E. and Wood, A.J.J., Influence of age and smoking on drug kinetics in man: studies using model compounds, *Clin. Pharmacokinet.*, 5:309–319, 1980.

29. Dollery, C.T., Fraser, H.S., Mucklow, J. C., and Bulpitt, C.J., Contribution of environmental factors to variability in human drug metabolism, *Drug Metab. Rev.*, 9:207–220, 2979.

30. Lieber, C.S., Interaction of ethanol with drugs and vitamin therapy, *Ration. Drug Ther.*, 19:1–7, 1985.

31. Iber, F.L., Drug metabolism in heavy consumers of ethyl alcohol, *Clin. Pharmacol. Ther.*, 22:735–742, 1977.

32. Vesell, E.S., Pharmacogenetics: multiple interactions between genes and environment as determinants of drug response, *Am. J. Med.*, 66:183–187, 1979.

33. Vessell, E.S., Genetic host factors: determinants of drug response, *N. Engl. J. Med.*, 313:261–262, 1985.

34. Bennett, W.M., Arnoff, G.R., Morrison, G.M., Golper, T.A., Pulliam, J., Wolson, M., and Singer, I., Drug prescribing in renal failure: dosing guidelines for adults, *Am. J. Kidney Dis.*, 3:155–193, 1983.

35. Reidenberg, M.M. and Drayer, D.E., Drug therapy in renal failure, *Annu. Rev. Pharmacol. Toxicol.*, 20:45–54, 1980.

36. Bircher, J., Altered drug metabolism in liver disease: therapeutic implications, in *Recent Advances in Hepatology,* Thomas, H.C. and Macsween, R.N.M. (Eds.), Churchill-Livingston, London, 1983, 101–113.

37. Williams, R.L. and Benet, L.Z., Drug pharmacokinetics in cardiac and hepatic disease, *Annu. Rev. Pharmacol. Toxicol.*, 20:389–413, 1980.

38. Morselli, P.L., Franco-Morselli, R., and Bossi, L., Clinical pharmacokinetics in newborns and infants: age-related differences and therapeutic implications, *Clin. Pharmacokinet.*, 5:485–527, 1980.

39. Green, T.P. and Mirkin, B.L., Clinical pharmacokinetics: pediatric considerations, in *Pharmacokinetic Basis for Drug Treatment*, Benet, L.Z., Massoud, N., and Gambertoglio, J.G. (Eds.), Raven Press, New York, 1984, 269–282.

40. American Association of Retired Persons, *Prescription Drugs: A Survey of Consumer Uses, Attitudes, and Behavior,* AARP, Washington, D.C., 1984.

41. Massoud, N., Pharmacokinetic considerations in geriatric patients, in *Pharmacokinetic Basis for Drug Treatment*, Benet, L.Z., Massoud, N., and Gambertoglio, J.G. (Eds.), Raven Press, New York, 1984, 283–310.

42. Greenblatt, D.J., Sellers, E.M., and Shader, R.I., Drug disposition in old age, *N. Engl. J. Med.*, 306:1081–1088, 1982.

43. McInnes, G.T. and Brodie, M.J., Drug interactions that matter — a critical reappraisal, *Drugs,* 36:83–110, 1988.

44. Ross, E.M., Pharmacodynamics: mechanisms of drug action and the relationship between drug concentration and effect, in *The Pharmacological Basis of Therapeutics*, Gilman, A.A., Goodman, L.S., Rall, T.W., and Murad, F. (Eds.), 7th ed., Macmillan, New York, 1985, 35–48.

45. Keirns, J.J. and Farina, P.R., Drug action and receptor theory, in *Modern Drug Research — Path to Better and Safer Drugs*, Martin, Y.C., Kutter, E., and Austel, V. (Eds.), Marcel Dekker, New York, 1989, 1–34.

46. Ganellin, C.R. and Durant, G.J., Histamine H_2-receptor agonists and antagonist, in *Burger's Medicinal Chemistry*, Wolf, M.D. (Ed.), John Wiley & Sons, New York, 3:487–552, 1981.

47. Chung, F.Z., Wang, C.D., Potter, P.C., Venter, J.C., and Fraser, C.M., Site directed mutagenesis and continuous expression of human beta-adrenergic receptors: identification of a conserved aspartate residue involved in agonist binding and receptor activation, *J. Biol. Chem.*, 263:4052–4055, 1988.

48. Fraser, C.M., Chung, F.Z., Wang, C.D., and Venter, J.C., Site directed mutagenesis of human beta-adrenergic receptors substitution of aspartic acid-130 by asparagine produces a receptor with high-affinity agonist binding that is uncoupled from adenylate cyclase, *Proc. Nat. Acad. Sci. USA*, 85:5478–5482, 1988.

49. Holmgren, J., Actions of cholera toxin and the prevention and treatment of cholera, *Nature*, 292:413–417, 1981.

50. Vaughan, M., Choleragen, adenylate cyclase, and ADP-ribosylation, *Harvey Lectures*, 77:43–62, 1982.

51. Gawler, D., Milligan, G., Spiegel, A.M., Unson, C.G., and Houslay, M.D., Abolition of the expression of inhibitor guanine nucleotide regulatory protein Gi activity in diabetes, *Nature*, 327:229–232, 1987.

52. Kenakin, T., Drug and receptors — an overview of the current state of knowledge, *Drugs*, 40(5):666–687, 1990.

53. Miller, D.D., Structure-activity relationship and drug design, in *Remington's Pharmaceutical Sciences*, 18th ed., Gennaro, A.R. (Ed.), Mark Printing Company, Easton, PA, 1990, 422–432.

54. Stewart, R.B., Adverse drug reactions, in *Remington's Pharmaceutical Sciences*, 18th ed., Gennaro, A.R. (Ed.), Mark Printing Company, Easton, PA, 1990, 1330–1343.

55. Faich, G.A., Knapp, D., Dreis, M., and Turner, W., National adverse drug reaction surveillance: 1985, *JAMA*, 257:2068–2070, 1986.

56. D'Arcy, P.F. and Griffin, J.P. (Eds.), *Iatrogenic Diseases*, 3rd ed., Oxford University Press, Oxford, 1986.

57. Jick, H., Miettinen, O.S., Shapiro, S., Lewis, G.P., Suskind, V., and Slone, D., Comprehensive drug surveillance, *JAMA*, 213:1455–1460, 1970.

58. Kramer, M.S., Leventhal, J. M., Hutchinson, T.A., and Feinstein, A.R., An algorithm for the operational assessment of adverse drug reactions. I. Background, description, and instructions on use, *JAMA*, 242:623–632, 1979.

59. Hutchinson, T.A., Leventhal, J. M, Kramer, M.S., Karch, F.E., Lipman, A.G., and Feinstein, A.R., An algorithm for the operational assessment of adverse drug reactions. II. Demonstration of reproducibility and validity, *JAMA*, 242:633–638, 1979.

60. Davies, D.M., *Textbook of Adverse Drug Reactions*, Oxford University Press, Oxford, 1985.

61. Moya, F. and Thorndike, V., Passage of drugs across the placenta, *Am. J. Obstet. Gynecol.*, 84:1778–1798, 1962.

62. Timiras, P.S., Course of pregnancy, early embryonic stages, and differentiation, in *Developmental Physiology and Aging*, Timiras, P.S. (Ed.), Macmillan, New York, 1972, 61–78.

63. Iams, J.D., and Rayburn, W.F., Drug effects on fetus, in *Drug Therapy in Obstetrics and Gynecology*, Rayburn, W.F. and Zuspan, F.P. (Eds.), Appleton-Century-Crofts, Norwalk, CT, 1982, 9–17.

64. Davies, D.M., Disorders of the fetus and infant, in *Textbook of Adverse Drug Reactions*, Davies, D.M. (Ed.), Oxford University Press, Oxford, 1985, 78–127.

65. Millstein, L.G. FDA's pregnancy categories, *N. Engl. J. Med.*, 303:706, 1980.

66. Committee on Drugs, American Academy of Pediatrics, Transfer of drugs and other chemicals into human milk, *Pediatrics,* 84:924–936, 1989.
67. Beeley, L., Adverse effects of drugs in later pregnancy, *Clin. Obstet. Gynecol.,* 13:197–214, 1986.
68. Briggs, G.G., *Drugs in Pregnancy and Lactation,* 3rd ed., Williams & Wilkins, Baltimore, MD, 1990.

4

DEVELOPMENT OF NEW DRUGS BY RESEARCH INSTITUTES AND THE PHARMACEUTICAL INDUSTRY

I. MEDICAL AND PHARMACEUTICAL RESEARCH IN DRUG DEVELOPMENT

Drug development is a complex process that integrates a broad range of multidisciplinary expertise. Medical and pharmaceutical research together provide a solid foundation for advanced drug development. The pharmaceutical industry's main production efforts focus on drugs or medical devices that have therapeutic application and can be broadly utilized by the health-care system. Successful outcomes begin with accurate predictions of market need. Applying accumulated knowledge and resources to plan future research programs requires a stepwise approach. If the etiology of a disease can be identified, studies can then begin to characterize the causative agent and define pathophysiologic mechanisms leading to disease outcome. This information provides a basic foundation for developing substances to prevent, treat, or, ideally, cure disease. When the etiology and/or mechanisms are unknown, highly specific therapeutic and prophylactic drugs are difficult to develop. Pharmaceutical research and development depend largely on cutting-edge science in areas that can improve current techniques, instrumentation, and our understanding of the mechanisms of disease processes.[1-3]

Many drugs are discovered as an incidental finding during other efforts to identify novel treatment methods. The traditional way to identify new drugs has been to screen a large number of natural products and synthetic chemical compounds for a desired effect. Even 50 years ago, drug materials were derived only from natural products. An example is menthol, isolated from peppermint and used for the treatment of coughs, colds, and pain. Recently, many more effective drugs have been isolated, identified, and produced from synthetic analogs. Although the screening process for new drugs successfully identifies new pharmaceutical agents and reduces laborious processes, screening does have limitations. The screening process requires an appropriate procedure to test large numbers of chemicals and to select active compounds. Initial screening may not immediately detect pharmacologic activity, and thus, an active structure might not be discovered promptly.

■ Screening tests in animal models might not be suitable to extrapolate effects on human disease. A chemical agent may be extensively metabolized to different compounds, which in humans might not be absorbed or distributed in active form.
■ Screening is a random, repetitious, and time-consuming process for identifying promising chemical agents.

When an active (lead) compound is identified and its chemical structure elucidated, modifying the basic molecular structure can improve pharmacological activity and diminish reactogenicity. For certain natural proteins, the gene itself may be manipulated so that organisms can directly synthesize protein molecules or a modified compound. For example, modifications of the original cephalosporins led to second- and third-generation products with broader spectra of antimicrobial coverage.[4]

An in-depth understanding of biochemical mechanisms makes it possible to design using pharmacodynamic and quantitative structure–activity relationship approaches. When the disease process is understood at a molecular level and target molecules are defined, drugs can be designed specifically to interact with a target molecule.

Drug discovery is both a culmination of new ideas and a reiterative process. Modification of active structures can improve specific pharmacological activity and lower toxicity. Decisions are based on repeated testing. Although great progress has been made to correlate chemical structure and activity, particularly for antimicrobial agents, there are still many diseases, including cancer, viral infections, cardio-vascular disease, and mental disorders, that need new, improved drugs. As more is understood about mechanisms of disease onset and progression, drug development can be transformed further from empirical screening to a more rational design.

Today, the structure of biochemical receptors and the mechanism of enzyme function are more clearly understood. Molecules that act as receptor agonists or antagonists or as enzyme inhibitors are prime targets for new candidate drugs. A homologous series of analogs illustrates how slight structural differences produced by sequential chemical changes in carbon chain length improve pharmacologic activity. Short alkyl chains frequently elicit low biological activity. As the chain length increases, activity peaks at an optimal chain length, then decreases as longer methylene groups are added.

Structure–activity studies involve the synthesis of molecular fragments within an active compound and assessment of subsequent pharmacological activity. This process is used when the structure is known and the molecule has a significantly novel therapeutic action. For example, cocaine has been used as a prototype molecule for developing more effective local anesthetics. The critical part of the molecule required for activity is the hydrophilic amine segment attached to an intermediate chain, which in turn is attached to a lipophilic ester function, e.g., procaine. The carbomethoxy group, or tropane ring, of cocaine is not required for its activity and can be removed, e.g., tropacocaine or ß-eucaine.

Another approach used in structure–activity relationship studies is to add functional groups to a molecule with known pharmacological activity. Replacement of the N-methyl group with the larger N-phenethyl group to form N-phenethyl normorphine produced a compound six times more potent than morphine. Precise stereochemistry is also important to determine optimal drug-target activity. For example, pentobarbital and amobarbital are positional isomers that differ only in the five-carbon side chain attached to the barbiturate ring system. Other strategies used in advanced drug design involve converting the conformation of a flexible molecule to a rigid molecule in order to define a spectrum of structure for optimal receptor binding, e.g., dopamine can exist in many conformations due to its side-chain carbon–carbon bond and thereby exhibit different biological activity.[5–7]

Quantitative structure–activity relationship (QSAR) studies are extensively applied to modify, design, and synthesize new molecular structures, as well as to consistently produce quantitative biological data.[8,9]

Computerized statistical and molecular modeling methods have rapidly facilitated extraction of useful information and provide a physical basis for meaningful interpretation of a multidimensional data matrix. The pKa values of substituted benzoic acids, and the ability to donate or withdraw electrons from the carboxyl group, can be predicted as a function of substituents attached to the ring. Essential biologic parameters required for drug activity can be incorporated into certain mathematical equations to predict a theoretical drug response. In a study of thyroxine derivatives, replacement of iodine by a t-butyl group was predicted to result in a more active molecule. Computer-generated scenarios reduce the likelihood that structure modification will result in a negligible response. QSAR and computer science techniques are routinely applied in pharmaceutical practice for new drug experimental design, data collection, correlation, statistical analysis, retrieval, modeling, and documentation.[10,11] Many approaches to drug design are based on the relationship of drug–receptor interaction. In the biosystem, many substrates are metabolized by enzymes. Drugs can act by altering the ability of the substrate to interact with the enzyme or receptor.

Metabolite antagonism, or antimetabolites, is also based on similar target-specific interactions. Antagonism is based on the principle that molecules shaped as mirror images of enzyme surfaces can inhibit enzyme function. An antimetabolite thus competes with a metabolite by blocking the active site on the enzyme surface. This type of model led to the design of the antiulcer drug, cimetidine, and its derivatives. Hypersecretion of histamine is known as a cause of excessive gastric hydrochloric acid production and associated ulceration formation. Classical antihistamines counteract histamine activity associated with allergies and hay fever, but not gastric hyperchlorhydria. Therefore, it is assumed that histamine acts on two different types of receptors. Receptors blocked by antiallergenic drugs are termed H1 receptors, while those involved with gastric acid secretion are designated as H2 receptors. The H1 receptor antagonists do not resemble histamine, but rather, contain molecular blocking groups that inhibit histamine access to the H1 receptor. The design of H2 receptor antagonists, however, does involve changes to the main structural portion of histamine. An imidazole ring carrying a basic side chain was lengthened, which resulted in a less acidic environment. Replacing a carbon on the imidazole ring, however, resulted in a more acidic environment. From several hundreds of synthesized compounds, cimetidine and rimantidine were eventually discovered as effective drugs for ulcer therapy.[12,13]

Advancements in the capacity of hormone, antibody, and drug antagonists have progressed at a rapid pace. A receptor is typically composed of proteins or glycoproteins consisting of a few subunits. Many receptors are distributed in cell membranes, with a hydrophobic end on the inside and a hydrophilic terminus on the outside. Receptors have been isolated, sequenced, cloned, and reconstituted from many sources. Their chemical structures have been studied extensively. More information, however, is needed to precisely correlate molecular structures within the active site with folded structures in final form, their function, and specific pharmacological response. Modification of biologic products is especially relevant to vaccine technology. The principle of immunization involves injecting a person with an inactivated pathogen, toxoid, or recombinant cell-surface antigen to induce a protective immune response without causing the disease. Active vaccination elicits long-lasting immunity through the formation of the memory B cells that rapidly generate antibodies. Defining protein structure–activity relationships, together with recombinant DNA and peptide synthesis, are considered the most innovative and promising contributions to drug design.

During FY 2001, seven new biological products were developed and licensed by the FDA for use in therapy (Table 1). More than 125 biotechnology products are currently in various stages of development. These products include vaccines, anticoagulants, colony-stimulating factors, erythropoietins, human growth hormones, interferons, interleukins, monoclonal antibodies, and tumor necrosis factors.[14,15] The hepatitis B vaccine (Recombivax HB, Merck Sharp & Dohme, 1986) was manufactured by recombinant DNA technology through the following procedures:[16]

1. Genetic material (DNA) is extracted from hepatitis virus.
2. The gene that directs production of surface protein antigen is identified and isolated from viral chromosomal DNA and inserted into a plasmid.
3. Plasmids that contain the specific gene are cloned into yeast cells.
4. Yeast cells are grown by fermentation to produce large amount of hepatitis surface protein.
5. After 48 hrs, yeast cells are ruptured to release surface protein antigen. The protein antigen is isolated and purified.
6. Preparations of surface protein antigen are combined with preservative and aluminum hydroxide adjuvant to form the final vaccine.

Biotechnology methods are fast becoming a powerful adjunct to traditional drug development. Almost every major pharmaceutical industry now uses biotechnology to develop drugs, vaccines, and biological products.[17,18]

II. CHALLENGES IN PRECLINICAL DRUG TESTING

Sometimes it seems easier for a camel to go through the eye of a needle than for a new molecular entity to be successfully developed, evaluated, and licensed for use. Drug development today is an extremely costly, long, and difficult endeavor. Yet, in the end, the journey of bringing forth a new drug through rigorous testing and the licensure process is exciting and rewarding work. Critical decision-making by scientists from multiple disciplines occurs throughout the process. Each pharmaceutical laboratory collaborates with development planning divisions to provide greater assurance that the process for developing effective and safe agents proceeds smoothly. From an industry standpoint, the general stages of drug development are shown as follows:[19]

1. Basic research — depends on new and original ideas. It is necessary to apply the current knowledge in basic medicine, pharmaceutical sciences, and biology.
2. Screening and identification — to synthesize new chemical compounds or isolate and purify active agents from natural substances.
3. Selection — to perform initial tests on pharmacological activity and toxicity.
4. Evaluation of drug safety — to assess short- and long-term toxicity; determine absorption, distribution, biotransformation, and excretion (ADME).
5. Pharmacological action and clinical trial — to assess drug effects in a series of clinical trials.
6. Manufacturing and pharmaceutic design — to plan large-scale manufacturing procedures and optimal pharmaceutical forms for drug delivery.

For a new drug to be developed, licensed, and eventually transformed into a useful therapeutic agent, it is imperative that research scientists and marketing management cooperate with each other; each unit understands and recognizes the role of the other. Success or failure of the drug development process depends equally on competent, cohesive group efforts.

Drug discovery usually begins with the need for a drug to fill specific demands in a therapeutic area or a particular clinical indication. Following identification and preliminary *in vitro* testing for pharmacological activity, decisions are made to terminate, modify, or select product candidates. Potential candidates undergo further chemical analyses, testing for safety, pharmacological action, drug metabolism, and then evaluation in clinical trials. The data from these tests in part fulfill regulatory requirements to ensure the safety and effectiveness of new drugs. Initial investigation by chemical analysis characterizes the compound's identity, potency, purity, and stability. After a chemical compound is isolated in a pure state, purity, elemental analysis, configuration, and structure are assessed. A number of sensitive and sophisticated instruments measure infrared absorption, mass, nuclear magnetic resonance, ultraviolet, and optical rotary dispersion. Physicochemical properties are examined by a series of tests that determine melting points, partition coefficient, dissociation constant, pKa, and decomposition profile. The stability of the new drug is then determined for both bulk and final container forms under accelerated conditions of heat, light, humidity, and storage time. These results provide supporting data that the drug is consistently manufactured exactly as intended.[20]

Pharmacological evaluation of a new chemical agent begins at discovery and extends throughout the development process. Results from *in vitro* receptor binding assays, enzymatic activity, and effect on cell culture provide an initial assessment of primary pharmacological effects. Once the desired pharmacological actions are determined by initial testing, a series of *in vivo* and *in vitro* tests are conducted to further study the mechanisms of action and possible adverse reactions on specific organ systems. These data are used to assess therapeutic effects as well as toxicity: Does the new agent have the desired pharmacodynamic effects? Does the chemical bind with strong affinity to the specific receptor? What is the magnitude of the dose–response relationship in normal and pathological animal models? Does a variable drug response occur among different species, strains, or individual animals? What is the effective dose and the therapeutic index of the compound?

Pharmacokinetic studies, which provide information about the rate and extent of absorption, distribution, biotransformation, and excretion, are vital to the development process.[21] The biotransformation of a drug is the major determinant of the intensity and duration of its pharmacological and adverse reactions. Weak radioisotopes, such as β-emitters carbon-14 (14C) or tritium (3H), are incorporated into metabolically stable portions of the molecule. Emitted signals enable quantifiable measurements of the parent drug and its metabolites. The primary objectives of these studies are to determine drug absorption, the duration of drug exposure, and the extent of drug metabolism. From comparison of blood levels and excretion data after oral and intravenous administration, a favorable compound is selected, based on maximal absorption (bioavailability based on the area under a serum drug concentration–time curve [AUC]), optimum pharmacokinetics (maximum concentration attained, Cmax; time to maximum effect, Tmax; half-life, $T_{1/2}$; and clearance), effective delivery to tissues (volume of distribution, Vd; protein binding), and route of elimination.

Toxicology studies are performed in animal species shown to have drug metabolism and disposition parameters approximately similar to those in humans. General guidelines for animal safety studies are usually provided to allow toxicologists some flexibility to tailor studies to a drug indication. In many cases, each drug is studied as a new and individual entity. Guidelines are not intended to prohibit investigators from exercising scientific judgment and expertise when designing a safety study. This point is particularly applicable to preclinical safety studies of recombinant DNA and hybridoma products.

The thalidomide disaster of the 1960s heightened public concern regarding the importance of animal studies to predict potential human malformations. Hence, much attention is paid to a drug's potential for interfering with reproductive processes. Accordingly, studies are aimed at evaluating drug effects on fertility, mating behavior, estrous cycles, conception rates, and uterine and placental function; on implantation, embryogenesis, and development; and on parturition and the newborn, lactation, weaning, physical growth, and behavior development of the offspring. Carcinogenicity studies are costly, complex, and time-consuming. Evaluating the selected route of administration and dosage occurs for most of the animal's life span. Which drugs should be tested for potential carcinogenicity? Currently there is no general agreement on this question. Drugs that are chemically related to known carcinogens, or that produce metabolites similar to known carcinogens, or that might damage rapidly dividing tissues, or that are intended for long-term or repeated use are candidates highly considered for carcinogenic testing.

Carcinogenicity testing in rodents is relatively crude, insensitive, and inefficient. Additional statistical analyses are often necessary to demonstrate a difference between the incidence of neoplasms in test rodents and those occurring spontaneously in control animals. Since testing extends for the majority of an animal's life span, rodent species with short longevity are usually selected. Rats, mice, and hamsters are species commonly used; more specifically, Sprague-Dawley, Wister, Long-Evans, and Fisher-344 rats, as well as CD-1 and B6C3F1 mouse strains, are most frequently employed. Dosage selection is one of the most difficult and complicated aspects of a carcinogenicity test. At present, the concept of the maximum tolerated dose (MTD) is applied. The MTD is determined by conducting a 90-day subchronic study in rats and mice using several dose levels and performing the appropriate clinical and pathological tests. MTD is defined by the National Cancer Institute as "the highest dose of the test agent given during the chronic study that can be predicted not to alter the animal's normal longevity from effects other than carcinogenicity." Thus, the MTD should be the highest dose that causes no more than a 10% weight decrease, as compared to control groups, and does not cause mortality, clinical signs of toxicity, or other pathologic lesions that would be predicted to shorten the animal's natural life span. Once the MTD has been determined, other doses may be set as fractions of it, e.g., MTD/2 or MTD/4. If a maximum tolerated dose response cannot be established in animals, the highest dose tested may be selected as 100 to 200 times the usual recommended therapeutic dosage. A thorough evaluation and accurate interpretation of animal toxicity is critical to decide whether plans to initiate clinical trials can proceed.

III. STRATEGIES AND PLANNING FOR CLINICAL TRIALS

Pharmaceutical research is a continuum that starts at basic research and extends to clinical investigation. Only a few new molecular entities studied in clinical trials will ever be developed and marketed, and even fewer of these marketed entities will generate profitable returns on initial investments.[22] Since clinical development is the most costly portion of drug development, pharmaceutical companies must carefully design and manage plans for clinical trials. Compounds have an increased chance of success if preclinical screening, safety tests, and clinical trials can be conducted in a reasonable timeframe.

Clinical development plans can be divided into strategic and operational segments. The strategic plan involves scientific and regulatory phases, in which the target and direction of the research program are defined. The operational plan addresses the approach and process to reach the ultimate goal of new drug development quickly and efficiently.[23]

The regulations that govern the use of an investigational drug at pre phases appear at 21 CFR 312. Under certain restricted conditions, an IND may be waived to treat patients with an investigational drug.

A. Phase I Trial — Safety and Early Clinical Pharmacology

The initial strategy for Phase I is to conduct a single-dose safety study in healthy volunteers. A 28-day tolerance and pharmacokinetic study in healthy volunteers is then conducted for long-term administered drugs. These studies provide preliminary safety information to support plans for an efficacy trial. The long-term Phase I trial includes investigation of biopharmaceutics, the dose proportionality using two dosage levels, bioavailability of the proposed formulation, and drug interactions.

Phase I studies not only provide an initial safety assessment, but are also the primary phase in which characterization of the drug's performance is made. A sponsor who intends to introduce a new drug to humans should submit an IND to the Center for Drug Evaluation and Research, where it is forwarded to one of the Medical Review Divisions in the Office of Drug Evaluation, I or II. Generally, the IND will be forwarded to the divisions with the most suitable clinical, pharmacology, and/or chemistry expertise to evaluate the product components and proposed indication. The FDA has 30 days from the date of receipt of the application to review the file and determine if the proposed clinical trial may proceed. If the sponsor has not been contacted by the 30th day, the study may proceed. However, if the agency has issued a clinical hold to delay the clinical study start date, the trial may not proceed until all concerns are adequately addressed. The following conditions may result in the imposition of a clinical hold:

- Subjects would be placed at an unreasonable risk of illness or injury.
- The clinical investigators are not qualified to perform the proposed trial.
- The investigator's brochure is misleading, erroneous, or incomplete.
- The application does not contain sufficient information to assess the risks to study participants.

Among these conditions, the most common reason for a clinical hold is the lack of sufficient information to determine that the proposed study can be performed safely.

Actions of drug metabolites in animals may not be reflective of potential toxicities in humans. If available, a suitable animal species should be chosen for toxicity testing. Data on plasma drug levels for both the parent drug and metabolite can be used to monitor the extent of drug exposure in clinical trials. Final study reports submitted in an IND include data from single-dose animal toxicity studies with a subsequent 1- to 3-month follow-up period.

The regulatory chemist is responsible for reviewing data that describe the identity, quality, purity, and strength of the investigational new drug. In Phase I, emphasis is placed on the identification and control of raw materials used in the synthesis of the compound. The IND application should contain the description of the drug substance and product including physical, chemical, and biological characteristics; the general method of synthesis or isolation; and limits of impurities.

The composition of the drug product, along with stability data, needs to support adequate product potency and stability for the duration of the clinical trial. Manufacturing information may be submitted to a regulatory agency in a separate file called a drug master file (DMF), which protects the need to release confidential proprietary manufacturing information to the IND sponsor. Frequently, an investigational drug is not manufactured by the IND sponsor; the sponsor must obtain a letter of authorization from the DMF folder that allows the regulatory agency to review the material in it.

B. Phase II Trial — Clinical Efficacy and Safety

Phase II trials consist of establishing the efficacy and long-term safety of a new drug. All safety aspects evaluated in Phase I studies are now extensively examined in a larger population. The objectives of a Phase II trial are as follows:

- To assess preliminary clinical efficacy and estimate incidence of adverse reactions in the target population
- To define an optimum therapeutic dose and dosing regimen
- To provide detailed pharmacokinetic and pharmacologic activity data to support plans for Phase III trials

Phase II studies evaluate dosing regimens, tolerability of the drug in the target population, additional pharmacokinetic parameters, and sensitivity of specific treatment outcomes. Adequate and well-controlled trials that are capable of demonstrating the effectiveness of a treatment are described in 21 CFR 314.126. There are several designs that can be considered to be adequate and well-controlled:

- Placebo concurrent control — patients are randomized to treatment with the test drug compared with a placebo.
- Dose comparison concurrent control — patients are randomized to receive one of several fixed doses of treatment. The goal is to show a correlation between the dose given and the treatment outcome.
- No-treatment concurrent control — these trials involve randomization to receive treatment or no treatment. This design is appropriate when the outcome measures and the effect from the placebo are negligible.
- Active-treatment concurrent control — patients are randomized to receive either a new drug or a drug known to be active for the intended clinical use.
- Historical control — all patients receive treatment and their outcomes are compared with results from a group of similar patients who have not received treatment. Historical control data are usually available from the literature.

Other important considerations for Phase II studies include selecting an appropriate outcome measure that is clinically relevant to changes in the disease state, easily measured during a specified timeframe, and quantitatively reflects changes in drug effect. The study duration must also be long enough to detect a drug effect. In some cases, long-term response is used to predict ultimate outcome and therapeutic effect. Data from Phase II trials enable further correlation of dose or plasma drug level with pharmacological response. While Phase II clinical trials are ongoing, more refined characterization of the drug substance and product is performed. Limits on impurities are defined further, and additional stability data are generated.

At the end of the Phase II trial, a conference with the FDA is usually scheduled to confirm the intended indication, review data from Phase II trials, and propose a Phase III trial plan. Agreements are sought on the following issues:

- Major disagreements arising from the submitted information for preclinical trials, clinical studies, and manufacturing procedures

- The need for additional studies to support results from existing preclinical pharmacokinetics, safety studies, and/or manufacturing procedures
- The accuracy of the claimed indications

With regard to the criteria that must be met for approval of a treatment indication, the FDA provides several guidance documents that outline important regulatory considerations to incorporate into the therapeutic development plan. These guidelines provide useful information to sponsors about standards for all three phases of premarketing development.

In addition, advisory committees can provide guidance to the FDA when controversial regulatory issues arise. At least one appointed committee is assigned to each review division. Appointment of committee members are made by the FDA commissioner; they serve tenures of 2 to 4 years. Advisory committees meet several times a year to discuss issues pertinent to the agency.

In late Phase II and early Phase III, pivotal trials are conducted; the results from these trials comprise the principal data used to support licensure approval. Scientists put forth great effort to review these protocols and identify problems that might complicate the analyses. Early review and open communication help reduce wasted time, effort, and resources, avoid designing clinical trials incapable of producing valid scientific information, minimize broad exposure to a large study population, and identify unnecessary risks incurred from an investigational treatment. Key study design issues for definitive trials are outlined below:

- Inclusion and exclusion criteria
- Dose regimens
- Methods of collection and timing of safety and effectiveness data
- Duration of treatment and follow-up assessment
- Identification of the primary outcome variables, their time of assessment, and statistical analysis
- The primary population to be included in the analysis

C. Phase III Trial — Large-Scale Clinical Studies

Data from early clinical trials provide a framework from which to plan large-scale studies. Based on the clinical pharmacology, therapeutic properties, and adverse reactions observed thus far, appropriate choices of endpoints, sample size, statistical methods, and efficacy analyses can be proposed for large-scale clinical studies. The main objectives of a Phase III trial are as follows:

■ To conduct large-scale safety assessments to fully characterize less common and serious adverse event rates
■ To evaluate the proposed dose and dosing regimen as intended for market use
■ To formulate conclusions about overall therapeutic efficacy and safety in the actual target population based on statistical methods

There is often overlap between the conduct of Phase II and Phase III trials. A Phase III study can begin before the completion of Phase II studies. All forthcoming data necessary to demonstrate safe and effective use of the product are collected and used to support approval of the intended indication. While a Phase III trial is ongoing, meetings may be arranged with regulatory agencies to discuss the format of clinical study reports, required documents needed for a complete drug application.

The pediatric population poses special challenges to evaluate mutagenic vulnerability, delayed toxicity, and different pharmacokinetics in clinical trials. Thus, decisions about the ratio of appropriate therapeutic benefit vs. tolerance for adverse reaction is frequently a concern. During lactation and initial physical development, an infant undergoes rapid physiologic and metabolic changes. During periods of rapid growth and development, infants and children may be particularly susceptible to adverse drug effects.

If a disease occurs primarily in the pediatric population, is rare and/or life-threatening, with no alternative therapy available, initial Phase I studies involving children may be considered. Usually, pharmacological evaluations are initially assessed in adults. The chronicity of disease also affects the timing of pediatric studies in the overall clinical development plan. If the disease is acute and short-lived, pediatric patients are evaluated in Phase I and II studies. When the disease is chronic, however, pediatric clinical trials are usually not conducted until Phase III. For drugs intended for extensive, long-term use, e.g., psychoactive drugs, special preclinical tests are conducted prior to clinical trials. Studies in pediatric patients should be planned so that effects of the test drug can be assessed during various stages of growth and development.

Vaccine products are different from other drugs in that they tend to produce a specific immune response and they are administered in small amounts only 1 to 3 times. In general, a Phase I vaccine study provides data primarily for safety, but also includes immunogenicity objectives to evaluate magnitude and duration of the immune response in the target population. The vaccine is the only type of biological product in which drug administration involves healthy individuals. For childhood vaccines, investigational products are usually assessed in adults or older children first, then evaluated in young children.

The frequency of local and systemic reactions is important. Common queries for adverse events include local erythema, swelling, pain, edema, fever, malaise, irritability, diarrhea, vomiting, and anorexia. Some events are unique to a specific type of vaccine, such as encephalopathy observed in infants receiving pertussis-containing vaccines. For inactivated vaccines, such as polio vaccine (Salk type) and toxoid bacterial vaccines, safety assessments focus on the potential for incomplete inactivation or reactivation following removal of the denaturant reagent. Likewise, live attenuated vaccines may revert back to the wild-type virulent strain during replication in the host.

Alternative strategies to demonstrate efficacy using immunologic endpoints or via an animal model have received much attention. Design of an efficacy trial showing cases of disease prevention may not be possible if a disease occurs at low frequency, if the disease is well controlled by previously licensed vaccines, or if it is ethically unacceptable (e.g., anthrax). At present, there is a trend toward harmonizing basic clinical trial design and regulatory requirements so the number of costly studies can be minimized. Studies conducted internationally, however, sometimes create additional complicated medical, technical, legal, and ethical issues.[24]

D. NDA Phase and Phase IV — Postmarketing Monitoring

When a sponsor believes it has obtained sufficient information to demonstrate safety and efficacy, an NDA is submitted to the FDA for market approval. The application contains detailed information on all aspects of clinical and preclinical development, product composition, and manufacturing procedures. If the submitted data and documentation meet regulatory requirements, the application is approved as early as 180 days after the application is submitted.

Monitoring of the safety and effectiveness of a drug does not end upon approval by the FDA. The FDA continues to monitor effectiveness of the drug, and possible latent-onset and rare adverse events. Sponsors of approved NDAs are still required to submit reports of adverse events that occur during the marketing period. Reported information includes correspondence from health-care practitioners, the published literature, or foreign marketing experience. A sponsor is required to report all serious and unexpected adverse events which are fatal or life-threatening, result in permanent disability, require hospitalization, or cause congenital abnormality, cancer, or overdose. An initial report must be submitted to the FDA within 15 days of the receipt of the information.

For newly approved drugs, sponsors should report adverse reactions quarterly for the first 3 years after the date of approval, and annually thereafter. Anyone can report an adverse event to the FDA or to a drug manufacturer. Since public reports are voluntary and not actively solicited, adverse event rates obtained from this source are often underestimated. Moreover, serious adverse reactions may not be reported. In an effort to monitor more accurate drug-related adverse events, a program called MedWatch was developed in 1993. This system was designed to encourage health-care providers to report adverse events and to make reporting these events a part of practitioners' professional responsibilities.

Drug development from discovery and synthesis in the laboratory, through preclinical tests and clinical trials, to licensure and eventual use in the market, is a costly, time-consuming, and complex enterprise. Frequent communication between regulatory agencies and the pharmaceutical industry is necessary to efficiently introduce safe and effective drugs to the public.

IV. PHARMACEUTICS AND THE DRUG DELIVERY SYSTEM

Pharmaceutics is an area of study involving drug manufacture, formulation, stability, and effectiveness. Therapeutic effect, especially for children, is highly dependent on compliance with recommended dosing regimens. While pharmaceutical products should primarily be stable, efficacious, easy to administer, and safe, pediatric drug compliance is largely associated with an attractive appearance and pleasant taste. Factors affecting presentation include the route of administration, physicochemical properties of the product, formulation, and drug concentration at the absorption site. A drug delivery system ideally enables controlled drug delivery rates to achieve optimal pharmacokinetic properties while also maintaining stability in variable physiologic conditions.

During the 1950s, sustained-release products appeared as a major class of drugs in which the duration of a drug's pharmacologic action was increased; thus reducing frequent dosing. During the 1960s and 1970s, controlled-release or site-specific drug delivery systems were introduced. These types of delivery systems further improved sustained drug action by improving bioavailability, efficacy, and delivery of the drug to a specific site of the body.[25,26]

Many drugs today rely first on the drug finding its way to the pharmacologic receptor, and second, on the body's own excretion mechanism magically preventing undesirable adverse effects. The concept of a site-specific delivery system offers a solution to these expectations. The site-specific delivery system uses a carrier, similar to a "magic missile," which directs active molecules to a specific body site. Upon reaching the site, the drug is released either passively or following a specific site-recognition event. In more scientific terms, targetable delivery systems depend either on their physicochemical interactions within the body, or on the guidance of the carrier to exert a therapeutic effect.

The mechanics of each drug delivery system take into account the duration and specificity of each treatment plan. In general, drug formulations using a specialized delivery system are anticipated to improve compliance by minimizing the number of daily doses needed. This concept applies to treatment of acute disease and long-term maintenance of medical conditions, such as hypertension and diabetes. Drugs utilizing a particular delivery system are anticipated to reach the site of action more directly, thus reducing or eliminating undesirable adverse reactions. With the technology present thus far, drug delivery systems have only partially achieved these goals.

Oral administration is, in practice, the most utilized route of administration due to its ease and acceptance by the patient. A delivery system that could be incorporated as part of many oral drug therapies would enable greater flexibility in dosage design. Prodrugs represent one such system; they utilize resident enzymes to regenerate the parent compound. Other factors to take into account include mechanisms for timed release of the active compound, penetration, and absorption through an epithelial membrane into the blood circulation. Factors that influence the oral sustained-release dosage formulation include the biologic half-life of the drug, absorption characteristics, metabolic activity, physicochemical properties of dose size, solubility, and stability.

Targeted delivery systems are frequently utilized in cancer therapies. Treatment is based on the following characteristics of malignant cells: (1) their biologic activities and surface properties interfere with a host's immune system recognition and elimination, which leads to progressive physiologic imbalance between tumors and their hosts; and (2) biochemical differences between tumor cells and host cells are frequently quantitative rather than qualitative. The basis for site-specific delivery systems in cancer chemotherapy takes into account that overproduction of a specific cell marker and rapid cell turnover are characteristic of tumor cells compared to normal host cells. By targeting drug delivery to a specific cell marker, uptake, distribution, and concentrate effect can be directed more toward tumor cells and less toward normal cells. The site-specific delivery system is comprised of three key stages:

1. Specific distribution of the dosage form through endothelial passage over a particular organ
2. Selective targeting to a specific pathologic part of the organ
3. Selective intracellular delivery of the drug

This delivery system approach has been used for both monolithic particles and lipidic molecules, such as liposomes. Liposomes are phospholipid vesicles whose size ranges from 50 nm up to several micrometers in diameter. A few drugs have been incorporated as specific ligands onto the surface of liposomes, such as desialylated fetuin,[27] glycoproteins,[28] and immunoglobulins.[29,30]

Pharmaceutical product stability is defined as the capacity of a drug formulation, when packaged in a specified container, to maintain its physical, chemical, and therapeutic specifications within acceptable limits. Assessment of drug stability starts from the date of manufacture and packaging of a formulated product. Chemical and pharmacologic activity and physical characteristics are measured up to the time when these properties are expected to deteriorate. More specifically, stability is the period during which claimed potency of the chemical and pharmacologic activity, and physical characteristics can be maintained. Expiration date is then defined as the period during which the product remains stable when stored under recommended conditions.

Factors influencing product stability include how labile the active ingredient is within the proposed formulation, the interaction between active and inactive ingredients, manufacturing process, the container, and shipment and storage conditions. Certain physical factors, such as heat, light, and moisture, may initiate or accelerate chemical reactions. Changes in physical appearance, e.g., color fading or haziness, are sometimes indications of decreased product stability. Discoloration itself variably affects therapeutic capacity, but often causes medical personnel and public consumers to lose confidence in the product. A cloudy solution or a separated emulsion may also lead to erratic absorption or distribution patterns. Likewise, routine assessments to minimize incompatible ingredients and chemical interactions, e.g., oxidation, reduction hydrolysis, and racemization are desirable.

Oxidation is a prime cause of drug product degradation. This type of reaction involves the addition of oxygen, removal of hydrogen, or the loss of electrons from an atom. Oxygen can be present in the air space within the pharmaceutical container or dissolved in the liquid vehicle itself. Drugs sensitive to oxidation can be prepared in a lyophilized formulation, packaged in sealed containers, and traces of oxygen replaced by an inert gas such as nitrogen. Oxidation is accelerated by increases in temperature and radiation, and also in the presence of a catalyst, such as a heavy metal. Less than 0.0001% concentration of cupric, ferric, or chromic ion greatly reduces the stability of penicillin, epinephrine, and procaine hydrochloride. Some chelating agents, such as calcium disodium edentate and ethylenediamine tetra-acetic acid (EDTA), are used to complex or bind the metal, making it chemically unavailable for participation in the oxidative process. Oxidation may be inhibited by the use of antioxidants. Electrons released by an antioxidant are accepted more readily by free radicals than by the drug product. Commonly used antioxidants for drugs formulated in an aqueous medium include sodium sulfite (Na_2SO_3), sodium bisulfite ($NaHSO_3$), ascorbic acid, and hypophosphorous acid (H_3PO_2). For oil-based media, ascorbyl palmitate, hydroquinone, α-tocopherol, butylated hydroxyanisole, and ascorbyl palmitate are utilized.

Hydrolysis also contributes to degradation of a drug product. Drugs containing an ester or amide linkage are easily hydrolyzed. Examples include meningococcal polysaccharide (a polymer with $\alpha2$–8 mannosamine phosphate as the repeating unit), cocaine, thiamine, and benzylpenicillin. The rate of hydrolysis depends on the temperature and the pH of the solution. A 10°C increase in the storage temperature usually doubles the rate of reaction. Accordingly, when hydrolysis occurs, the concentration of the active ingredient decreases proportionally to the amount of degraded product. Excipients are selected to help stabilize the active compound. Buffers are included in the final formulation when small changes in pH are anticipated to cause major degradation of the active ingredient; pH is a critical factor in determining the rate of hydrolysis since many hydrolysis reactions are catalyzed by hydronium and hydroxyl ions. The amount of moisture present likewise can profoundly affect the rate of hydrolysis. If a reaction is accelerated by water, other solvents, such as glycerin, propylene glycol, or alcohol can be used instead. The stability of meningococcal polysaccharide vaccine, for instance, is improved when lactose is added as a stabilizer to remove residual moisture.

Methods used to ensure product sterility against bacteria include autoclaving liquid preparations at 121°C under 15 pounds of steam pressure for 20 minutes, or passing the liquid through a small-pore filter (0.22- or 0.45-µm). In addition, preservatives are often added to liquid and semisolid formulations, especially ophthalmic and injectable preparations. Antimicrobial agents are added to reduce risks of contamination with mold, yeast, and bacteria. A preservative provides greater assurance that product sterility will be maintained during storage until the time of use. Bacteriostatic agents are contraindicated for dextrose-containing intravenous solutions and plasma substitutes. These products are typically prepared in large volumes (500 to 1000 ml), and the amount of preservative needed to adequately reduce bacterial growth in such a large volume itself would cause an adverse reaction. Preservatives are, however, well tolerated in small-volume parenteral solutions. The preservatives commonly used in pharmaceutical preparations include benzoic acid (0.1 to 0.2%), sodium benzoate (0.1 to 0.2%), ethanol (0.1 to 0.2%), phenol (0.1 to 0.5%), thimerosal (0.002 to 0.01%), phenylmercuric nitrate and acetate (0.002 to 0.01%), benzalkonium chloride (0.002 to 0.01%), and a combination of methylparaben and propylparaben (0.1 to 0.1%).

To ensure the efficacy, safety, and purity of pharmaceutical products, the FDA enforces compliance with the requirements of Good Manufacturing Practice (GMP) regulations. The first GMP regulations were issued in 1963. Since then, they have been revised periodically. An outline of these regulations is shown in Table 9.[31]

V. REGULATORY ISSUES INVOLVED IN PLANT MEDICINES[32–34]

Plant medicines (e.g., herbal products, Chinese traditional medicines, and Kampo drugs) have been used in Asia and other areas of the world for many years. Recently, plant-derived products have been the subjects of increased attention. A few plant compounds exhibit possible therapeutic effect against allergy symptoms, cancer, AIDS, and chronic degenerating diseases.[35,36] Since these compounds are typically used as dietary supplements, rather than as drugs or biological products, regulations for the approval of therapeutic indications are currently evolving. Evaluation of quality, efficacy, safety, purity, stability, and consistency of potential plant medicines has not been done. In many cases, the claims included in the package insert of plant medicines are based on limited observations and anecdotal experience, rather than

Table 9   The Outline of Current Good Manufacturing Practice (GMP) Regulations

A. General provisions
1. Scope
2. Definitions

B. Organization and personnel
1. Responsibilities of quality control unit
2. Personnel qualifications
3. Personnel responsibilities
4. Consultants

C. Buildings and facilities
1. Design and construction features
2. Lighting
3. Ventilation, air filtration, air heating and cooling
4. Plumbing
5. Sewage and refuse
6. Washing and toilet facilities
7. Sanitation
8. Maintenance

D. Equipment
1. Equipment design, size, and location
2. Equipment construction
3. Equipment cleaning and maintenance
4. Automatic, mechanical, and electric equipment
5. Filters

E. Control of components and drug product containers and closures
1. General requirements
2. Receipt and storage of untested components, drug product containers, and closures
3. Testing and approval or rejection of components, drug product containers, and closures
4. Use of approved components, drug product containers, and closures
5. Retesting of approved components, drug product containers, and closures
6. Rejected components, drug product containers, and closures
7. Drug product containers and closures

F. Production and process controls
1. Written procedures; deviations
2. Charge-in of components
3. Calculation of yield

-- continued

Table 9 (continued)   The Outline of Current Good Manufacturing Practice (GMP) Regulations

4. Equipment identification
5. Sampling and testing of in-process materials and drug products
6. Time limitations on production
7. Control of microbiological contamination
8. Reprocessing

G. Packaging and labeling control
1. Materials examination and usage criteria
2. Labeling issuance
3. Packaging and labeling operations
4. Tamper-resistant packaging requirements for over-the-counter human drug products
5. Drug product inspection
6. Expiration dating

H. Holding and distribution
1. Warehousing procedures
2. Distribution procedures

I. Laboratory controls
1. General requirements
2. Testing and release for distribution
3. Stability testing
4. Special testing requirements
5. Reserve samples
6. Laboratory animals
7. Penicillin contamination

J. Records and reports
1. General requirements
2. Equipment cleaning and use log
3. Component, drug product container, closure, and labeling records
4. Master production and control records
5. Batch production and control records
6. Production record review
7. Laboratory records
8. Distribution records
9. Complaint files

K. Returned and salvaged drug products
1. Returned drug products
2. Drug product salvaging

From Lee, C.J., *Development and Evaluation of Drugs from Laboratory through Licensure to Market*, CRC Press, Boca Raton, FL, 1993. With permission.

biochemical analyses, studies in suitable animal models, or controlled clinical trials.

Since many botanical products are currently used in the U.S. as dietary supplements, these products are subject to regulations for this general indication. Under the Dietary Supplement Health and Education Act of 1994 (DSHEA), a dietary supplement may be advertised and sold only for the following purposes:

■ To alleviate a nutritional deficiency
■ To affect a structure or function of the human body
■ To maintain such structure or function

Products approved as a dietary supplement cannot claim to diagnose, treat, cure, or prevent any disease without undergoing appropriate evaluations for these indications. Without sufficient data, statements promoting a therapeutic, prophylactic, or diagnostic indication would be misleading.

Drug development plans for a botanical product vary depending on the intended indication. If data are intended to support U.S. market approval as an over-the-counter (OTC) drug, an OTC drug monograph would be submitted to the FDA. Similarly, if an indication for treatment of disease is sought, a new drug application (NDA) is submitted.

Botanical drugs are commonly isolated from complex mixtures that contain poorly defined chemical constituents. In many cases, the active ingredient has neither been identified, nor the pharmacological activity well characterized. Therefore, the chemistry, manufacturing, and controls (CMC) documents are necessarily different for botanical drugs than for purified chemical drugs. General considerations for assessing manufacturing procedures and drug components may likewise differ. Conventional outcome measures for purity, potency, safety, and consistency might be more meaningful if assessed by spectroscopy, chromatography, chemical and biological assays, quality control of raw materials, manufacturing in-process controls, and process validation.

Previously approved botanical products available in the U.S. for an OTC indication might be eligible for consideration in the OTC drug monograph system. For these products, data for safety and effectiveness, including results of adequate and well-controlled clinical studies, would be supported by information in the published literature.

A botanical product evaluated for a therapeutic indication requires an IND application. For botanicals approved in accordance with DSHEA, additional CMC and toxicological data required to initiate a clinical trial are likely to be minimal relative to requirements for a novel product. Similar to drugs and biologic products, previous results from international studies can be used to support initial clinical studies in a U.S. population. Clinical evaluation of botanical drug products for safety and effectiveness does not differ significantly from evaluation of purified chemical drugs.

Plant materials used in manufacturing botanical drug products frequently are not characterized, have variable composition, and often contain contaminants. Thus, careful attention to quality control results for plant raw materials and in-process control tests during manufacturing and validation process for the final product is important. A single formulation and a uniform dosing regimen should be consistent throughout the clinical evaluation. If possible, a single batch of botanical product should be processed from the same starting material. Sufficient quantities should also be available for evaluation in pivotal clinical trials.

Information for the final formulation should describe the product composition, recommended dose and dosing regimen, route of administration, and a statement that the product has not been adulterated with potent, toxic, purified chemical drugs, biotechnologically modified, or combined with other naturally derived drugs.

Sound regulations for plant medication research and development, clinical evaluation, manufacturing process, and quality control would ideally provide a structured process for market approval as therapeutic products and further acceptance by the Western medical community.

REFERENCES

1. Burger, A., Drug design, in *Drug Development,* Hamner, C.E. (Ed.), CRC Press, Boca Raton, FL, 1982, 53.
2. Martin, Y.C., Kutter, E., and Austel, V. (Eds.), *Modern Drug Research: Paths to Better and Safer Drugs,* Marcel Dekker, New York, 1989.
3. Clarks, C.R. and Moos, W.H. (Eds.), Drug design, in *Drug Discovery Techniques,* John Wiley & Sons, New York, 1990, 1.
4. Newall, C., Injectable cephalosporin antibiotics: cephalothin to ceftazidime, in *Medicinal Chemistry — The Role of Organic Chemistry in Drug Research,* Roberts, S. and Price, B. (Eds.), Academic Press, London, 1985, 209.
5. Daniels, T.C. and Jorgensen, E.C., Physicochemical properties in relation to biological action, in *Wilcon and Gisvold's Textbook of Organic Medicinal Chemistry and Pharmaceutical Chemistry,* 8th ed., Doerge, R.F. (Ed.), Lippincott, Philadelphia, 1982, 5.
6. Nogrady, T., Receptor-effector theories, in *Medicinal Chemistry, A Biochemical Approach,* 2nd ed., Oxford University Press, New York, 1988, 58.

7. Miller, D.D., Structure-activity relationship and drug design, in *Remington's Pharmaceutical Sciences,* 18th ed., Gennaro, A.R. (Ed.), Mark Printing Company, Easton, PA, 1990, 422.

8. Blankley, C.J., Introduction: a review of QSAR methodology, in *Quantitative Structure–Activity Relationship of Drugs,* Topliss, J.G. (Ed.), Academic Press, New York, 1983, 1.

9. Martin, Y.C., Other mathematical methods of use in quantitative structure–activity studies, in *Quantitative Drug Design,* Marcel Dekker, New York, 1978, 233.

10. Lien, E.J., QSAR in medicinal chemistry: an overview, *Chinese Pharm. J.,* 42, 93, 1990.

11. Kollman, P., Molecular modeling, *Annu. Rev. Phys. Chem.,* 38, 303, 1987.

12. Rogers, E.F., The antimetabolite concept in drug design, *Annu. Rev. Med. Chem.,* 11, 233, 1976.

13. Burger, A., Drug design, in *Drug Development,* 2nd ed., Hamner, C.E. (Ed.), CRC Press, Boca Raton, FL, 1990, 39.

14. Pharmaceutical Manufacturers Association, Biotechnology medicines in development, *Gene. Engin. News,* 12 (January), 27, 1992.

15. Dibner, M.D., The impact of biotechnology on the pharmaceutical industry, in *Drug Development,* 2nd ed., Hamner, C.E. (Ed.), CRC Press, Boca Raton, FL, 1990, 241.

16. Hilleman, M.R., Present and future control of human hepatitis B by vaccination, in *Modern Biotechnology and Health: Perspectives for the Year 2000,* Patarroyo, M.E., Zaabriskie, J.B., and Pizano-Salazar, D. (Eds.), Academic Press, Orlando, 1987, 199.

17. Sykrybalo, W., Emerging trends in biotechnology: perspective from the pharmaceutical industry, *Pharm. Res.,* 4, 361, 1987.

18. Marderosian, A.H., Biotechnology and drugs, in *Remington's Pharmaceutical Sciences,* 18th ed., Gennaro, A.R. (Ed.), Mark Printing Company, Easton, PA, 1990, 1416.

19. Lee, C.J., Ishimura, K., Nakajima, T., and Huang, J.T., New drug development and good laboratory practice (GLP) in the United States, *Lab. Animal Sci. Technol.,* 2, 95, 1990.

20. Kesterson, J.W., Preclinical drug discovery and development, in *Clinical Drug Trials and Tribulations,* Cato, A.E. (Ed.), Marcel Dekker, New York, 1988, 17.

21. Sheiner, L.B. and Benet, L.Z., Premarketing observational studies of population pharmacokinetics and new drugs, *Clin. Pharmacol. Ther.,* 38, 481, 1985.

22. Cato, A.E., The challenge of the clinical development of drugs, in *Clinical Drug Trials and Tribulations,* Cato, A.E. (Ed.), Marcel Dekker, New York, 1988, 1.

23. Cloutier, G. and Cato, A.E., Overall clinical drug development planning, in *Clinical Drug Trials and Tribulations,* Cato, A.E. (Ed.), Marcel Dekker, New York, 1988, 51.

24. Ackerman, S.K., Biological products in phase I and phase II clinical trials, in *Clinical Drug Trials and Tribulations,* Cato, A.E. (Ed.), Marcel Dekker, New York, 1988, 173.

25. Grass IV, G.M. and Robinson, J.R., Sustained- and controlled-release drug delivery systems, in *Modern Pharmaceutics,* Bander, G.S. and Rhodes, C.T. (Eds.), Marcel Dekker, New York, 1990, 635.

26. Tomlinson, E., Site-specific drug delivery using particulate systems, in *Modern Pharmaceutics,* Bander, G.S. and Rhodes, C.T. (Eds.), Marcel Dekker, New York, 1990, 673.

27. Gregoriadis, G. and Neerunjun, E.D., Homing of liposomes to target cells, *Biochem. Biophys. Res. Commun.,* 65, 537, 1975.

28. Juliano, R.L. and Stamp, D., Lectin-mediated attachment of glycoprotein-bearing liposomes to cells, *Nature,* 261, 235, 1976.

29. Gregoriadis, G., Meehan, A., and Mah, M.M., Interaction of antibody-bearing small unilamellar liposomes with target free antigen *in vitro* and *in vivo, Biochem. J.,* 200, 203, 1981.

30. Weissman, G., Bloomgarden, D., Kaplan, R. et al., A general method for the introduction of enzymes, by means of immunoglobulin-coated liposomes, into lysosomes of deficient cells, *Proc. Natl. Acad. Sci. U.S.A.,* 72, 88, 1975.

31. *Code of Federal Regulations,* Current good manufacturing practice for finished pharmaceuticals, Title 21, Part 211, FDA, Rockville, MD, 1990, 76.

32. Lee, C.J., Immunomodulating polysaccharides in plant medicine, in *Managing Biotechnology in Drug Development,* CRC Press, Boca Raton, FL, 1996, 120–126.

33. Mitscher, L.A., Pillai, S., and Shankel, D.M., Some transpacific thoughts on the regulatory need for standardization of herbal medical products, *J. Food Drug Anal.,* 8 (4):229–234, 2000.

34. Center for Drug Evaluation and Research, Guidance for industry botanical drug products, CDER, Food and Drug Administration, Rockville, MD, 2001, 1–48. http://www.fda.gov/cder/guidance

35. Otsuka, Y. Pharmacotherapy in oriental medicine, in *Recent Advances in the Pharmacology of Kampo (Japanese Herbal) Medicines,* Hosoya, E. and Yamamura, Y. (Eds.), Excerpta Medica, Tokyo, 1988, xvii-xxi.

36. Lee, C.J. and Lu, C.S., Studies on immunomodulating herbal polysaccharides, in *Professional Frontiers in the 21st Century,* Chinese–American Professionals Association of Metropolitan Washington, D.C., 2002, 3.32–3.42.

5

CHALLENGING PROBLEMS IN THE FUTURE

Health is not merely the absence of pain or disease, it is a state of sound physical, mental, and social well-being. The status of a person's health is thus a sustainable balance of responses that involves physiological, psychological, and environmental factors. The interaction between internal bodily defense mechanisms and external environmental influences are merely shifts in the continuum between illness and health.

In 1982, the U.S. Department of Health and Human Services (HHS) initiated proposals for national health goals and specific health objectives to prevent and reduce risks of developing heart disease, cancer, and the other major causes of death and disability. In response to an increasingly health-conscious America, the Department of HHS recommended the following lifestyle changes as part of an overall plan to prevent major disease: (a) the elimination of cigarette smoking, (b) adoption of a more nutritious diet, (c) reduction of alcohol consumption, and (d) establishment of an environment more conducive to healthy living.[1] Disease prevention efforts occurred at several levels of the health-care system. Primary prevention included generalized health promotion as well as specific protection against disease, such as balanced nutrition, environmental sanitation, and specific immunization. Secondary prevention emphasized early diagnosis and prompt treatment to halt the disease process and limit possible disability. Such measures included screening examinations for selected diseases and timely medical intervention to reduce the frequency of complications. Tertiary prevention promoted restoration and rehabilitation from diseases to prevent complete disability. Assistance in recovering enough to function in society, within the constraints of the disability, was also emphasized.[2]

I. PURSUIT OF A HEALTHY AND HAPPY LIFE IN AN AGING SOCIETY

Since the beginning of the 20th century, the prevalence of elderly individuals in the U.S. has been steadily increasing. In 1900, there were approximately 3 million persons 65 and older, which represented 4% of the total population. In 1965, the year Medicare and Medicaid were started, the number of elderly had increased to 18.5 million people, which was equivalent to 9.3% of the total population. In 1980, there were 25 million elderly individuals, which amounted to over 11% of the total population. The elderly population in the years 2000 and 2030 are estimated at 31 million and 46 million, which would comprise 12% and 17% of total population, respectively.[3]

At present, individuals aged 65 years are expected to live an average of an additional 16 years. Of this population, the ratio of elderly women to men who are 65 years old is 69 men per 100 women, but at 85 years of age, the ratio decreases to 44 elderly men per 100 elderly women. Thus, future medical problems and health-care provisions will necessarily need to accommodate elderly women more than elderly men. Financial security and health are perhaps the two most challenging problems facing the elderly today. The majority of this population is anticipated to have fixed incomes and to be living alone. From a physical health standpoint, the elderly are prone to develop memory deficits, decreased visual acuity and hearing, and diminished muscle strength. Likewise, metabolic disturbances, infection, and chronic health conditions might be more common. Hence, changes in the structure of the current health-care system are largely to prepare for the needs of an increasingly aged population.

There has been a substantial change in the etiology of health problems today as compared to the 1800s and early 1900s. Acute infectious diseases were the major cause of death in the early part of the 19th century, whereas chronic conditions, heart disease, cerebrovascular pathogenicity (stroke), and cancer are the major causes today. The advent of antibiotics and improved biotechnology has contributed largely to the treatment and prevention of infectious diseases. Efforts toward the diagnosis and treatment of acute disease, however, which were so successful in the past, are no longer the antidotes to today's challenges. As people are living longer, the focus of the health-care system will be more on early screening and preventive health measures. In addition, it is to be hoped that early interventions related to changes in biochemical mechanism, environmental factors, and lifestyle all will reduce the incidence of current major chronic health conditions

II. ASPECTS OF CURRENT BIOMEDICAL RESEARCH

A. Vaccine Development for Prevention of Infectious Diseases

During the early 20th century, the threat of infectious disease appeared to be receding. Major public health achievements included improved sanitation measures, prevention of childhood diseases through immunization, and the discovery of antibiotics. Drugs were hailed as miracle agents for the treatment of bacterial diseases. Enormous efforts focused on identifying new chemotherapeutic agents to treat pathogenic microorganisms. Mortality from infection, commonplace in the 19th century, was no longer a frequent occurrence in industrialized nations.

However, as it turned out, celebrated optimism occurred too soon. Pathogens developed a remarkable ability to evolve, adapt, and acquire resistance to chemotherapeutic agents in an unpredictable and dynamic manner. Today, new microbial threats are appearing in significant numbers, and diseases previously thought to be under control are re-emerging. The epidemic of acquired immunodeficiency syndrome (AIDS) led to a subsequent rise in reported tuberculosis (TB) cases; both diseases are quite prevalent in the U.S. In fact, a resurgence of infectious diseases, including multidrug-resistant TB, as well as high incidences of encapsulated bacteria, malaria, and cholera have occurred worldwide.

In the U.S., Lyme disease, Legionnaires' disease, hantavirus pulmonary syndrome, and West Nile viral encephalopathy are recent newly emerging diseases. Other emerging threats include diarrheal disease caused by toxigenic strains of *Escherichia coli*, and multidrug-resistant bacteria causing ear infections, pneumonia, and meningitis.

Immunization constitutes an important key method available for disease prevention. Vaccines provide both individual protection against life-threatening diseases and/or serious sequelae. Some vaccines also provide community protection by reducing transmission of pathogenic agents. If a sufficiently high proportion of the population is immunized, the disease transmission could be interrupted, which thus benefits the entire group. Protective herd immunity contributed to successful global elimination of smallpox and partial eradication of poliomyelitis.

Encapsulated bacteria are primary causes of serious disease among infants, the elderly, and immunocompromised persons. Despite antibiotic treatment, the mortality and morbidity from bacteremia, meningitis and pneumonia caused by these organisms are still high in these populations. The polysaccharide (PS) antigens contained in vaccines in the past, however, were poorly immunogenic and did not induce protective immunity in children younger than 18 months.

1. Glycoconjugate Vaccines[4-6]

The need to improve protective immunity in populations at highest risk resulted in the development of glycoconjugate vaccines. The coupling of polysaccharide (PS) antigens to a carrier protein overcame the immunologic limitations encountered with PS vaccines. The conjugation of *Haemophilus influenzae* type b (Hib) PS to diphtheria toxoid, tetanus toxoid, or mutant diphtheria protein CRM_{197} and subsequent vaccination with such glycoconjugate vaccine successfully resulted in a more than 97% reduction of Hib disease in Europe and the U.S. Using the same carrier proteins contained in the Hib conjugate vaccines led to the development of meningococcal bivalent conjugate and 7-valent pneumococcal conjugate vaccines.

Bivalent meningococcal vaccine, which includes serogroups A and C oligosaccharide conjugated to CRM_{197}, has been developed by Chiron Corporation (Italy) and evaluated in 90 toddlers in southern California. After two doses, serum bactericidal titers to serogroup A and C were approximately 20 and 300 times higher in children who received the conjugate vaccines than in those who received tetravalent groups A, C, Y, W-135 PS vaccine. Similar meningococcal serogroup A and C conjugate vaccines are being developed by Wyeth–Lederle and Aventis Pasteur, Inc. Meningococcal conjugate vaccines may reduce nasopharyngeal carriage of vaccine serogroups, which in turn, could reduce transmission to susceptible children through herd immunity.

In the U.S., *Streptococcus pneumoniae* causes an estimated 3000 cases of meningitis, 50,000 cases of bacteremia, and 7 million cases of acute otitis media annually. In young children, pneumococcus is the most common cause of bacterial meningitis. Although the 23-valent PS vaccine is efficacious in healthy adults, it is poorly immunogenic in children younger than 2 years of age. Prevnar™, a 7-valent pneumococcal conjugate vaccine manufactured by Wyeth–Lederle Vaccines, was licensed in 2000 in the U.S. for use in infants and toddlers. Vaccine efficacy against pneumococcal serotype-specific invasive disease was demonstrated in a study conducted in northern California that involved 37,000 infants. Protection against clinically diagnosed otitis media and pneumonia were also evaluated. At the time of the final efficacy analysis, 97% efficacy against pneumococcal serotype-specific invasive disease was shown in children immunized at 2, 4, 6, and 12 to 15 months of age.

The efficacy of the *Salmonella typhi* Vi PS vaccine was evaluated in Nepal and South Africa. In Nepal, the overall efficacy was 72% for blood culture–confirmed cases of typhoid fever at 20 months following vaccination. In South Africa, the efficacy was 50 to 61%. In 1994, Vi PS vaccine was approved in the U.S. for use in adults and children 2 years or older. *S. typhi* Vi PS conjugated to tetanus toxoid, diphtheria toxoid, or cholera toxin are significantly more immunogenic than a vaccine containing Vi PS alone. Clinical trials of Vi conjugate vaccines are ongoing. Development of other glycoconjugate vaccines for encapsulated pathogens, including Group B *streptococcus, Escherichia coli* O157, *Klebsiella pneumoniae,* and *Pseudomonas aeruginosa,* are also in various stages of clinical development.

Protective immunity to infection caused by encapsulated bacteria is improved by methods that enhance an antibody response to a specific capsular PS. Glycoconjugate vaccines produced by coupling a PS to a protein carrier have enabled infants and young children to produce protective antibody levels through a T-cell-dependent mechanism. The antibody response after immunization with a conjugate vaccine is quantitatively and qualitatively different from that observed with a PS vaccine. The successful production of Hib and 7-valent pneumococcal conjugate vaccines will lead to the development of effective conjugate vaccines for protecting against infection caused by other encapsulated pathogens.

2. DNA Vaccine[7–10]

Although the success of vaccination is well recognized, many conventional vaccines were developed to elicit humoral responses to viruses and bacteria. Immunization against intracellular organisms, however, such as human immunodeficiency virus (HIV), tuberculosis, malaria, and leishmania, requires cell-mediated protective immunity. Novel vaccine approaches are needed. One of the most promising approaches to solving this problem is the development of DNA (or genetic) vaccines. This type of vaccine contains the gene for a specific antigen, which results in both humoral and cellular immune responses.

DNA vaccine consists of a foreign gene for the desired antigen; the gene is cloned into a bacterial plasmid. Plasmid DNA, a small ring of double-stranded DNA derived from bacteria but unable to produce an infection, is engineered for expression in eukaryotic cells. The plasmid also frequently contains a bacterial antibiotic resistance gene, e.g., ampicillin or kanamycin resistance gene, and a promoter, e.g., from cytomegalovirus (CMV) or simian virus 40, for optimal expression in mammalian cells. The vaccine is usually delivered intramuscularly by a gene gun, which can deliver plasmids into skin cells or mucous membranes. After entering the cells, some of the recombinant plasmids make their way to the nucleus and instruct the cell to synthesize the encoded antigenic proteins. These proteins leave the cell and are taken up by antigen-presenting cells (APS, e.g., macrophages). Protein molecules are broken into fragments to interact with MHC (major histocompatibility) class I or II molecules. After such processing, the complexes are displayed on the cell surface and bind to Th cells. The activation of Th cell helps to elicit humoral (antibody-type) and cellular (killer-type) immunity (Figure 6).

DNA immunization provides several advantages over current vaccines:

- DNA vaccines mimic the effects of live attenuated vaccines in their ability to induce MHC class I restricted CD8+ T-cell response.
- DNA vaccines are relatively inexpensive to manufacture. They are easy to design and to produce in large quantity using recombinant DNA technology.
- They are as stable as other vaccines and can be stored with relative ease, eliminating the need for a cold chain.
- They can be engineered to carry genes from different strains of a pathogen to provide immunity against several strains at once.

Some researchers are testing vaccines composed of RNA, which leads to synthesis of encoded proteins. However, RNA is less stable than DNA. RNA vaccines have been studied much less extensively than DNA vaccines.

In addition to the components described above, DNA vaccines also contain specific nucleotide sequences that play an important role in the immune response of these vaccines. Synthetic oligodeoxynucleotides (ODNs), with sequence patterns that mimic those observed in bacterial DNA, were found to activate natural killer cells to secrete γ-interferon. More recently, it was shown that a specific

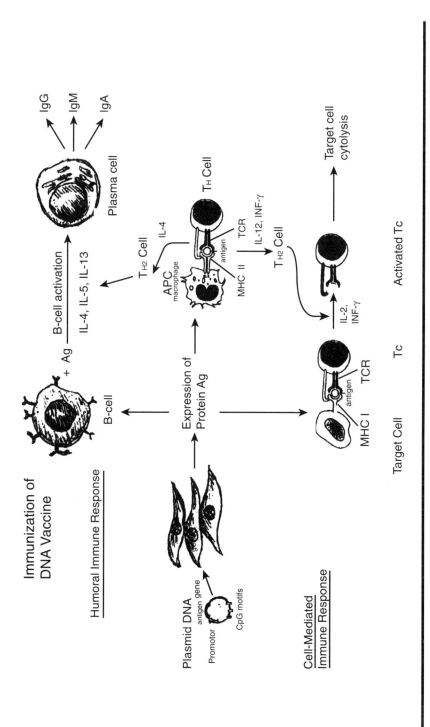

Figure 6   Immunization of DNA vaccine. APC, antigen presenting cell; Tc, cytotoxic T lymphocyte; MHC I, major histocompatibility complex class I; TCR, T cell receptor; MHC II, major histocompatibility complex class II.

sequence motif present in bacterial DNA elicited immune responses characterized by the production of interleukin (IL)-6, IL-12, tumor necrosis factor (TNF)-α, IFN-γ, and IFN-α. This motif consists of an unmethylated cytidine–phosphate–guanosine (CpG) dinucleotide. CpG motifs activate B cells to proliferate or secrete antibody. In addition, they enhance antigen-presenting cells (APCs), such as macrophages and dendritic cells, to secrete cytokines. Natural killer cells are indirectly activated by CpG motifs through cytokines induced by APCs. These cells are also stimulated directly or indirectly by CpG motifs.

Plasmid DNA induces the most potent immune response when CG sequences are flanked by two purines, adenine or guanine, to their C side and two pyrimidines, thymine or cytosine, to their G side.[7] In mice, plasmids containing these immunostimulating sequences induced a more vigorous antibody response and greater cytotoxic T-cell activity than did an otherwise identical vaccine. Therefore, increasing the number of CpG motifs in plasmids might amplify the immunogenicity of the antigenic codes in a DNA vaccine. Furthermore, for inducing an optimal effect, genes for signaling molecules called cytokines are incorporated into antigen-carrying or separate plasmids. For example, granulocyte-macrophage colony stimulating factor (GCSF), released from the cells of the immune system, stimulates the proliferation of antigen-presenting cells. Inclusion of the gene GCSF has been shown to stimulate overall responses to DNA vaccines.

In mice, investigators have found that helper T-cells called Th1 CD4+ cells secrete cytokines, e.g., IFN-γ that favor cell-mediated response, whereas other helper cells (Th2 CD4+ cells) secrete cytokines, IL-4, IL-5, and IL-13, which favor humoral immunity. A DNA vaccine including genes for HIV antigens and for IL-12 (Th1 cytokine) reduced production of anti-HIV antibodies in mice and markedly enhanced the response of cytotoxic T-cells to HIV antigens. It was found that the presence of IL-12 facilitates differentiation toward a Th1 response, whereas the presence of IL-4 results in Th2 differentiation.

The predominant Ig isotype generated following immunization with a gene gun is IgG1 (Th2 response), whereas after intramuscular immunization, the predominant Ig isotype generated is IgG2a (Th1 response). A plausible explanation for the observed Th2 response after vaccinating with a gene gun is that plasmid DNA is directly delivered into cells, thus bypassing surface interaction with CpG motifs. CpG motifs are present in the plasmid backbone and stimulate APCs to release Th1-type cytokines.

The potential of DNA vaccines to influence CD4+ T-helper cell responses has several practical applications. The ability of DNA vaccines to generate Th1 responses is useful for preventing disease caused by intracellular pathogens, e.g., TB, HIV, and leishmania, by inducing a CD8+ cytotoxic T-lymphocyte (TCL) response. In addition, a Th1 response generated by DNA immunization may prevent or limit an ongoing Th2 response, e.g., in asthma or allergic diseases.

DNA vaccines can induce a strong antibody response to protein antigens in mice, nonhuman primates, and humans. Moreover, the antibody response produced by plasmid DNA is protective in several *in vivo* animal models. In plasmid DNA-encoding influenza hemagglutinin antigen, the antibody responses peaked and reached a plateau between 4 and 12 weeks after a single DNA immunization in mice. Furthermore, antibody production increased in a dose-responsive manner following either a single injection or multiple injections of DNA. Antibody subtypes induced by DNA vaccines include IgG, IgM, and IgA. Antibody responses following DNA vaccination more closely resemble reported responses observed after natural infection. Similar antibody kinetic profiles provide an advantage over conventional protein vaccines.

Several safety concerns have been raised regarding the use of DNA vaccines, which include the following possible adverse reactions:

- DNA integration into the host genome, thereby increasing the risk of malignancy
- Response against transfected cells, and, in turn, the development of autoimmune disease
- Induction of immunologic tolerance and/or stimulation of cytokine production that alters the host's ability to respond adequately to other vaccines

Although plasmid DNA can persist at the site of injection for many months, to date there is no clear evidence that plasmids integrate into the host genome to cause malignancy.[11] Concerns that DNA vaccines may induce the development of autoimmune diseases arise from the immunostimulatory activity of CpG motifs in the plasmid backbone. To examine the possibility of autoimmunity, B cells secreting autoantibodies were studied in normal mice repeatedly immunized with a DNA vaccine. Shortly after vaccination, the number of IgG anti-DNA-secreting cells rose by two- to threefold. Increased cell number was accompanied by a 35 to 60% increase in serum IgG anti-DNA antibody titer. The rise in autoantibody level did not, however, result in the development of disease in normal mice or accelerate disease in lupus-prone animals.[12] Thus, although a theoretical possibility of autoimmune disease exists, results available in the currently published literature indicate that the level of autoantibody production elicited by DNA vaccines is not sufficient to cause disease manifestations. Hundreds of human volunteers have been exposed to plasmid DNA vaccines without serious adverse effects.

Because the immune system in an infant is immature, exposure to foreign antigens places the newborn at risk for developing immunologic tolerance. Factors influencing the development of neonatal tolerance include the antigen nature, concentration, age of the host, and mode of antigen presentation to the immune system. A DNA vaccine encoding a malaria circumsporozoite protein was found to induce tolerance rather than immunity in newborn mice. Neonatal mice treated with this vaccine were unable to generate T- or B-cell responses when treated with *Plasmodium yoelii* circumsporozoite protein (PyCSP) as adults, and thus were still susceptible to infection.[13,14] In this study, the induction of tolerance was dependent on the age at which the vaccine was given. Tolerance was observed only when vaccine was administered to mice younger than 8 days old. Efforts are under way to improve the overall immunogenicity of DNA vaccines by coadministering plasmids encoding cytokines or costimulatory molecules. These approaches can improve antibody responses in neonates and the elderly. Further investigations are needed to examine the possible adverse reactions and long-term safety caused by DNA vaccination.

DNA vaccines have initiated a new era of biomedical research by providing a powerful means to develop novel vaccines and immunotherapies. Several investigational DNA vaccines are currently being evaluated in clinical trials. Further studies are needed to overcome the issues of safety concerns as well as technical challenges of improving delivery systems and efficacy so that low-dose DNA vaccines can effectively prevent disease.

3. Edible Vaccine[15–17]

Recently, biotechnology has been applied to plants as a means to produce protein therapeutic agents and vaccines. Traditionally, bacteria such as *Escherichia coli* are used to produce recombinant proteins. These proteins predominantly exist in a denatured state and are partially or completely folded with mismatched disulfide bonds. Because of the complexities of producing proteins in bacteria, eukaryotic cells, e.g., yeast, and mammalian cells, were explored as possible alternative vectors to express recombinant proteins. Transgenic plants, compared to eukaryotic cells, are preferred for production of protein products. Plants have the capability to express foreign genes from a wide variety of sources, including viral, bacterial and other plant species. In addition, plants have the ability to perform complex post-translational modifications, e.g., glycosylation, and can produce relatively higher yields of expressed protein (exceeding 1% of total plant protein).

In early 1990s, the Children's Vaccine Initiative (CVI) encouraged investigation and development of oral vaccines to induce mucosal immune responses against pathogens invading mucosal surfaces. Vaccines eliciting this type of response might be more effective in treating or preventing respiratory disease, gastrointestinal infection, sexually transmitted diseases, and otitis media. The CVI also proposed goals to develop multicomponent vaccines and heat-stable vaccines for convenient use and distribution, particularly for developing countries. Use of transgenic plants was one approach to produce the desired protein antigens within an edible vector.

Plant vaccines, like subunit products, include selected antigens but contain no genes to construct whole pathogens. Thus the safety profiles are relatively comparable. Plant vaccines, however, do not require purification or refrigeration, and this helps to reduce overall cost. Currently, two major approaches are used for gene transfer into plants. One approach uses *Agrobacterium tumefaciens,* a naturally occurring soil bacterium capable of mobilizing a portion of the plasmid DNA into a plant cell. The other approach utilizes a device that accelerates penetration into plant cells by DNA-coated gold particles; this delivery system enables DNA to be integrated into the nuclear genome. The plant cells are then exposed to an antibiotic, such as kanamycin, to kill cells that lack the introduced genes; growth indicates that the antibiotic-resistant marker and the desired DNA were transferred successfully. The gene-altered cells then multiply and form a clump (callus). The callus later develops shoots and roots. The gene-modified plant is placed in soil to perpetuate growth and consequent protein antigen expression.

At present, antigens from hepatitis B virus (HBsAg), enterotoxigenic *E. coli* (heat-labile enterotoxin, LT-B), and Norwalk virus (Norwalk virus capsid protein, NVCP) have been successfully synthesized from transgenic tomato and potato plants. Alternatively, antigen-containing fruits fed to test animals were found to induce mucosal and systemic immune responses that protected the animals following subsequent challenge of the pathogens. The thick plant cell outer wall also serves as a protective coating to keep the antigens from being digested by gastric secretions. Once in the intestine, the cells gradually release the antigens.[16,17]

The ultimate question to be answered is whether plant vaccines can produce protective immunity in people. Healthy volunteers who ate peeled, raw potatoes containing the *E. coli* toxin B subunit gene demonstrated both mucosal and systemic immune responses.[15,16] Immune responses were also induced in 19 of 20 people who ate a potato vaccine containing Norwalk virus gene.[17a,b] Lettuce containing a hepatitis B antigen was fed to three volunteers; two individuals produced a high antibody response. Clinical trial and animal study results thus far indicate that plant vaccines are immunogenic and capable of eliciting protection against disease.

Several obstacles still pose barriers to developing an effective vaccine for human use:

■ *Selection of plant cells for gene expression.* Plants used to produce an edible vaccine should fulfill biotechnological requirements for gene transfer and distribution; fruits or vegetables used to produce childhood vaccines should be palatable to young children; and edible vaccines are desired in plants that can withstand high ambient temperatures or not require refrigeration. Plant species considered desirable expression systems for edible vaccines include bananas and tomatoes. Bananas need no cooking and can easily be grown in developing nations. A single banana contains about 1 to 1.5 g of protein. Taking into account an anticipated yield of 0.1 to 0.01% foreign protein expression per transgenic plant, each banana could produce 1 to 10 mg of recombinant protein. The protein antigen yield is equivalent to 1 to 10 conventional vaccine doses. Other plants under consideration are lettuce, carrots, potato, beans, and rice.

■ *High yield of protein antigen production.* Linking a gene to a constitutive promoter can increase protein expression. Activating the promoter to stimulate the gene expression can maintain sufficient antigen production. Sometimes, plants grow poorly when they produce large amounts of protein. Linking antigen genes with regulatory molecules can cause the genes to activate only at a selected time, such as after a plant is nearly fully grown, or only in its edible portions.

- *Effective vaccine delivery.* Adjuvants, e.g., LT-B, improve targeted vaccine delivery and resultant antibody responses. In addition, immune modulating factors, such as cytokines, co-expressed in plants, can enhance overall vaccine immunogenicity.
- *Suppression of immunity to antigens in food.* Oral tolerance to certain protein antigens can cause the body to diminish or suppress its responses to these antigens. The factors that lead to oral tolerance probably relate to antigen solubility and frequent exposure to the mucosal immune system. To develop edible vaccines, manufacturers should ensure that an antigen administered orally will not suppress immunity.

B. Resurgence in Search for Plant Medicines

Plant medicines (traditional Chinese medicines, herb products, Kampo medicines, botanical dietary supplements) have been used for thousands of years to relieve symptoms and cure disease. Over the past decade, plant medicines have become a topic of increasing global importance due to potential biomedical and economic implications. In the U.S., annual retail sales of botanical products increased from $200 million in 1988, to an estimated 5.1 billion in 1997, and consumer use of these products has increased by 380% in the past 10 years. The World Health Organization suggests that 65 to 80% of the populations in developing countries depend on traditional and botanical medicines as a primary source of health care.[18,19] Currently, traditional Chinese medicine (TCM) in China includes 30,000 TCM-related enterprises, 12,807 TCM varieties, domestic annual sales of 13.4 billion RMB in 1995, and was established as one of the important national goals of modernization during the period 1996 to 2005.[19a]

Plant medicine formulations usually comprise a mixture of several materials. Pharmacological investigations have focused on chemical substances contained in herbs. As a result, many useful compounds have been identified, and some have been used as ethical drugs. However, the methodological difficulties involved in characterizing combined herb formulations resulted in less acceptance by the Western medical community.

Since components contained in herbal medicines are not well characterized, adverse reactions due to active ingredients or excipients are difficult to determine. The mechanisms of GI absorption and metabolism during disease conditions are enormously complex. Consequently, clearly defined mechanisms are extremely difficult for plant medicines, even if studies are limited to the active ingredients.

1. Studies on Metabolism of Plant Medicines — Kampo Glycosides Are Natural Prodrugs

Kampo medicine consists of several combined herbs and is administered by the oral route. As ingested components pass through the gastrointestinal tract, they are metabolized by the intestinal flora and absorbed into the blood. Some components are directly absorbed, detoxified in the liver, excreted into the bile to interact with intestinal flora for biotransformation, and reabsorbed (Figure 7). Since water-soluble herb glycosides are poorly absorbed in the intestine, the glycosides have prolonged contact with intestinal flora. Thus, glycosides are less bioavailable and, consequently, might not exhibit the intended pharmacological activity. Several approaches have been proposed for the metabolism and interactions of herb components:

- Alterations of the chemical structure of the ingredients by saliva, gastric juice, bile, pancreatic juice, and intestinal bacteria
- Changes induced by hepatic drug-metabolizing enzymes
- Binding of active ingredients to their receptors and to plasma albumin
- Changes in the chemical structure and concentration of active ingredients in the blood and excretion into the urine, bile, and feces

Experimental results show that most ingested glycosides are resistant to gastric acid and digestive enzymes, and pass unabsorbed through the upper intestinal tract. Glycosides are retained in the lower GI tract, which is inhabited by thousands of anaerobic bacteria. There, they are mostly hydrolyzed by intestinal bacterial glycosidases to the corresponding aglycones, which are then absorbed slowly and continuously to exhibit pharmacological activities. Using germ-free and gnotobiotic rats to assess the role of human intestinal bacteria, it was demonstrated that glycosides are natural prodrugs; conversion to the active drug occurs specifically by intestinal anaerobe β-glycosidases. The following examples illustrate this point.

Glycyrrhiza root is an herb used in more than 70% of Kampo formulations. The active ingredient in glycyrrhiza root is glycyrrhizin, which exhibits anti-inflammatory, antiallergic, antiviral and steroid-like activities, and is widely used in herbal remedies. In addition, glycyrrhizin is 150 times sweeter than natural sugar, and thus is used extensively as a food additive.

1. Mouth — Oral administration.
2. Stomach — The ingested components pass through GI tract.
3. Intestine — Metabolized by enzymes of intestinal flora, absorbed into blood circulation, and excreted into feces.
4. Liver — Metabolized by enzymes in liver and excreted into bile.
5. Bile
6. Kidney — Active ingredients in the blood are excreted into the urine.

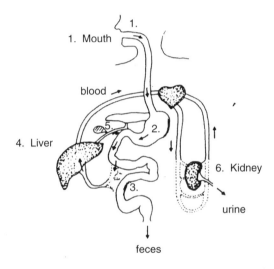

Figure 7   Metabolism of Herbal Products in Humans (Modified from Hosoya, E., Scientific reevaluation of Kampo prescriptions using modern technology, in *Recent Advances in the Pharmacology of Kampo* (Japanese Herbal) *Medicines*, Hosoya, E. and Yamamura, Y. (Eds.), Excerpta Medica Ltd., Tokyo, 1988.)

Eubacterium sp. GLH, an anaerobic bacterium isolated from human feces, metabolizes glycyrrhizin to glycyrrhetic acid via the enzyme glycyrrhizin β-glucuronidase. A summary of the metabolic process and resulting metabolites appears in Figure 8. Metabolism in rat and human livers corresponds to biotransformation of glycyrrhizin to an active metabolite. Rising circulating concentrations of glycyrrhetic acid were observed, with subsequent associated decreasing levels of glycyrrhizin. The inhibitory effect of glycyrrhetic acid on β-hydroxy steroid dehydrogenase, an enzyme that converts androstenedione to testosterone, is nine times greater than that of glycyrrhizin *in vitro*. These results

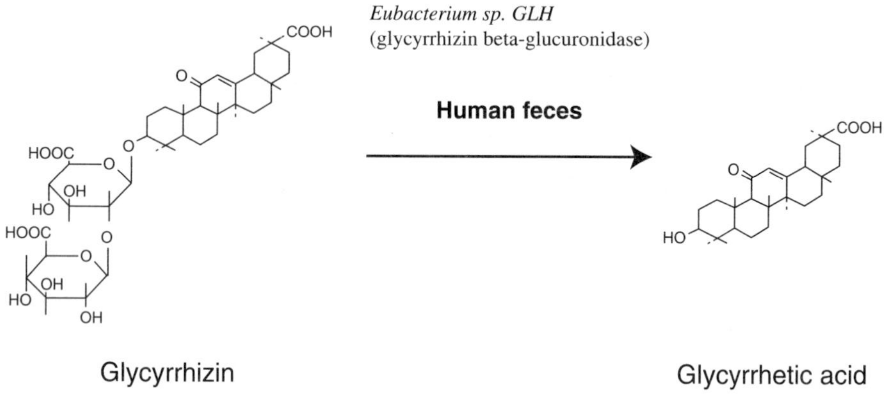

Figure 8 Hydrolysis of Glycyrrhizin by Glucuronidase Produced by Intestinal Flora (Modified from Kobashi, K., Glycosides are natural prodrugs — evidence using germ-free and gnotobiotic rats associated with a human intestinal bacterium, *J. Trad. Med.*, 15:1–13, 1998.)

suggest that primarily glycyrrhetic acid, rather than glycyrrhizin, induces the actions of *Glycyrrhizae radix in vivo*.

Baicalin is the main ingredient of scutellaria root (*Scutellariae radix*), which exhibits antiallergic and bile secretion stimulating activities. Baicalin is hydrolyzed human and animal β-glucuronidase to form an aglycon, baicalein. The circulating concentration of baicalin, however, which was measured as baicalein glucuronide, was higher than baicalin in the starting material. It was concluded that baicalin is not directly absorbed; rather, baicalin is metabolized by the intestinal flora, and absorbed as baicalein. Baicalein is reformed into baicalin and transferred into the blood circulation (Figure 9). Studies indicate that oral ingestion is essential for eliciting the pharmaceutical properties of Kampo medicine. Furthermore, individual differences in pharmacological effects might be due to differences in intestinal microbial composition.[20,21]

2. Immunomodulating Herbal Polysaccharides

Herbal polysaccharides have been reported to possess immunostimulating, antitumor, anticoagulative, antiemetic, and hypoglycemic activities.[22] The pharmacological activities of glycans and mannans isolated from the lentinan of *Lentinus edodes (Hsiang-ku)* and *Ganoderma tsugae* (Ling-chih) depend not only on the primary structure but also on conformation and micelle structure. The β(1→3) linkage of the

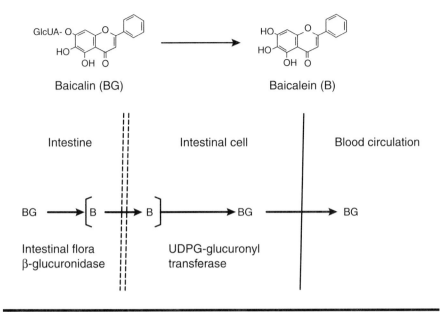

Figure 9   Absorption of Baicalin (BG) through the Metabolite Baicalein (B) (Modified from Kobashi, K., Glycosides are natural prodrugs — evidence using germ-free and gnotobiotic rats associated with a human intestinal bacterium, *J. Trad. Med.,* **15:1–13, 1998.)**

main chain in lentinan and pachymaran polysaccharides demonstrates strong activity against Sarcoma-180. Pusturan (GE-3), which contains a β(1→6) structure, also exhibits strong antitumor activity. The main immunostimulating polysaccharides in herbal medicines are shown in Table 10.

The mechanisms of immunostimulating and antitumor activities of plant polysaccharides are thought to involve functions related to phagocytosis amplification, macrophage activation, T-lymphocyte and alternative complement pathway activation, and enhancement of cell-mediated immune responses.[23] Immune responses naturally diminish with age. Since immunomodulating polysaccharides can enhance immune responses, they would be helpful in reducing susceptibility to disease.

New sources of biochemically active polysaccharides have attracted great attention, and subsequent demand for therapeutic immunostimulating therapies for immunodeficient diseases is increasing. Juzen-Taiho-To (JTT) has been administered to patients with anemia, anorexia, or general fatigue associated with postsurgical recovery, chronic disease, or childbirth. Observed clinical improvement indicates that

Table 10 Immunomodulating Polysaccharides in Herbal Products

Herb	Scientific Name	Active Components	Main Activity
Angelicae 當歸	Angelica sinensis A. acutiloba A. radix	PS (AR-arabinogalactan IIa) AR-4 IIa, AR IIb-1, AR IIb-2c PS AIP	Anticomplement activity
Astragalus 黃耆	Astragalus mongholicus Radix astragali A. membranaceus	Polysaccharide (PS) F3	Intensifies phagocytosis of immune system; restored hematopoietic function Stimulation of bone-marrow haematopoiesis
多瓜 柴胡	Benincasa cerifera Bupleurum falcatum	BCM BR-5-1	Activation of T lymphocytes Anti-complementary activities
Cnidii 川芎	Cnidium rhizoma C. officinale	PS Cnidirhan AG	Stimulation of cytokine production
Condyceps 蟲草	Condomopsis ophioglossoides C. tangshen	Saponins, PS	Enhances phagocytosis of macrophages
Ganoderma 靈芝	Ganoderma lucidum	PS (G-A)	Enhances immune functions; antitumor activity
Ginseng 人參	Panax ginseng	Ginsenosides Panaxosides Panaxatrial PS	Enhances phagocytosis of macrophages; promotes lymphocytic transformation; hematopoietic function

Herb	Scientific Name	Active Components	Main Activity
五加皮	Eleutherococcus senticosis	Eleutherosides PS	
豬苓	Grifola umbellata	GU-2	Antitumor activity
Hoelen 茯苓	Poria coccos	PS Pachymaran	
Lentinus 香菇	Lentinus edodes	PS	Enhances immune functions
	Coriolus versicolor	PSK	Stimulation of cytokine production; colony stimulating factor, IL-1
	Microellobosporia grisea	MGA	Tumor necrosis factor-α
Polyporus 豬苓	Polyporus umbellatus	PS (GU-2) (GU-3, GU-4)	Immunostimulating activity; anticancer activity
太子參	Pseudostellaria heterophylla	PH-1	Stimulation of cytokine production; TNF-α Stimulation of bone-marrow hematopoiesis
Tricholmataceae 菌花	Schizophyllum commure	Schizophyllan	Stimulation of IL-2 production
Zu sun (Kinugasatake) 竹蓀	Dictyophora indusiata	T-4-N (glucan) T-5-N (glucan)	Antitumor activity against sarcoma 180

PH-1, *Pseudostellaria heterophylla* fraction I; AIP, angelica immunostimulating PS; PSK, Polysaccharide K; BCM, *Beincasa cerifera* mitogen; F3, Fraction 3; MGA, *Microellobosporia grisea* anti-tumor PS; GU-2, *Grifola umbellata* fraction 2.

From Lee, L., Studies on immunostimulating herbal polysaccharides, in *Professional Frontiers in the 21st Century*, Chinese-American Professionals Association of Metropolitan Washington, D.C., 2002. With permission.

Table 11 Components of Juzen-Taiho-To

1.	*Astragali radix*	黄蓍	3.0 (gm)
2.	*Cinnamoni cortex*	桂皮	3.0
3.	*Rehmanniae radix*	地黄	3.0
4.	*Paeoniae radix*	芍藥	3.0
5.	*Cnidi rhizoma*	川芎	3.0
6.	*Angelicae radix*	當歸	3.0
7.	*Ginseng radix*	人參	3.0
8.	*Hoelen*	茯苓	3.0
9.	*Glycyrrhizae radix*	甘草	1.5
10.	*Atracylodis lancear rhizoma*	蒼朮	3.0

Target group: Recuperation after surgery or chronic diseases, exhaustion, fatigue, loss of appetite, paleface, dry skin, anemia, night sweat, dry mouth.

Indications: Weakness due to various diseases, tiring easily, exhaustion, loss of appetite, night sweat, cold hands and feet, anemia, KI-deficiency.

From Terasawa, K., *Kampo — Japanese-Oriental Medicine, Insights from Clinical Cases*, K.K. Standard McIntyre, Tokyo, 1993, 217.

JTT enhances immune responses and improves the function of the hematopoietic system. JTT consists of 10 component herbs (Table 11).

Data from Japanese studies show that JTT enhanced phagocytosis and mitogenic activity against spleen B cells, reduced mitomycin C side effects, and activated C3 complement and macrophages. TJ-48, a spray-dried powder of JTT extract, enhanced antibody, interleukin-2 (IL-2), and granulocyte-macrophage colony-forming cell (GM-CFC) production, as well as complement activating and mitogenic activities.[22]

Polysaccharides (PSs) have been isolated from the herbs *Angelicae radix* and *Hoelen*, which are two ingredients contained in JTT. *Angelicae* and *Hoelen* polysaccharides enhanced the PS IgG and IgM antibody responses to pneumococcal type 9V PS-protein conjugate, and caused rapid bacterial clearance from blood after challenge with virulent pneumococci. These plant PSs also stimulated TNF-α and INF-γ production, as well as IL-2 and IL-4 production. These results suggest that a possible protective mechanism involving plant PSs against bacterial glycoconjugate immunogens is through enhanced cytokines and immune responses. Incorporating plant PSs in conventional bacterial glycoconjugate vaccines may provide an alternative formulation for preventing pneumococcal disease.[24]

3. Growing Interest in Alternative Medicine

An increasing number of people worldwide are using complementary and alternative medicine (CAM) therapies. Perceived therapeutic effect is largely based on anecdotal cultural experience rather than quantitative and objective biomedical approaches. The increasing popularity of CAM therapies reflects a global change in general needs and values. Possible factors influencing a search for alternative health-care options include a rise in the prevalence of chronic disease, rapid and convenient access to global health information, reduced tolerance for adverse reactions caused by chemical drugs, and costly conventional health care.

In the U.S., use of one or more alternative medicines increased from 33.8% in 1990 to 42.1% in 1997. Although insurers and managed care organizations are increasingly considering coverage, patients pay billions of dollars for CAM therapies. Increased use of CAM has made it imperative that these topics be included in medical education.[24a] Alternative therapies used most often included herbal medicine, massage, megavitamins, energy healing and homeopathy for chronic back pain, anxiety, depression, and headache. Also in 1997, an estimated 15 million adults took prescription medications concurrently with herbal remedies and/or high-dose vitamins. Estimated expenditures for professional alternative medicine services increased 45.2% between 1990 and 1997; costs in 1997 were approximately $21.2 billion, with at least $12.2 billion paid out-of-pocket. This amount exceeded the 1997 out-of pocket expenditures for all U.S. hospitalizations.[25]

At present, tremendous resources are being allocated to understand and objectively study alternative health-care practices. Sixty percent of medical schools now include alternative medicine in their curricula; hospitals are establishing complementary and integrated medicine programs; and biomedical research institutes are conducting more studies to learn about these practices. Although efforts to characterize the therapeutic effects of complementary and alternative medicine are essential, the potential risks of alternative medicine must also be examined for the following reasons:

■ Alternative medicine practitioners lack in-depth and extensive professional training compared with training for conventional medical practitioners. Standardized testing and certification are also lacking.

■ The quality of many therapies has not been scientifically evaluated or continually monitored prior to general use. Lack of properly designed and conducted randomized controlled clinical trials is a major deficiency.

Physicians, pharmacists, and health-care personnel with increased science-based knowledge and familiarity about alternative medicines are better able to inform their patients of possible therapeutic benefits and limitations. Evaluation of any medical therapy, whether Eastern or Western, unconventional or mainstream, is best characterized by data from standardized, scientifically objective investigations.[26,27]

In the past, the natural health products industry has kept its distance from medical research and from clinical practice, and instead focused on short-term marketing advantages, e.g., obviating herbal products from required FDA review of efficacy, safety, and purity. An ideal approach would be for the natural products industry to work with biomedical research and FDA, so that consumers and health-care personnel could be better informed of potential harmful effects and assured with greater confidence that claimed health benefits actually exist. Although increased use of complementary and alternative medicine may continue, responses to general public demand will eventually draw attention to the need for reliable, scientifically based evidence of therapeutic effectiveness and safety. Therapeutic indications sought for alternative therapies and natural health products pose future challenges. Resolution of these challenges, however, will only be accomplished through collaborative industry scientific and regulatory efforts.

C. Recombinant Biotechnology and Gene Therapy

Recombinant DNA technology has led to the development of effective vaccines and therapeutic agents, and improved the quality of agricultural products. This technology enables transgenic expression of pigment genes to produce extravagant flowers with exotic shapes and colors. Recombinant growth hormones have practical applications to agriculture, resulting in leaner animal meat, improved milk production, and more efficient feed utilization. Transgenic plants and animals can also increase efficient production of protein molecules and medical therapeutics. The success of these efforts relies on continued research studies to understand the molecular mechanism of regulatory genes involved in biological processes.

Investigators have been interested in using plants as a system for the production of heterologous proteins. Production of a protein drug by peptide synthesis or cell cultures is an extremely expensive process. On the other hand, plants are easy to grow and large amounts of protein could be isolated. To date, various laboratory studies have been conducted to test the ability of different species to express proteins. These expression systems could provide a means to produce large quantities of human serum albumin and mouse monoclonal antibodies, or could be used as models for studying plant antitoxin therapy and herbicides.

Recombinant DNA technology was initially applied to manufacture recombinant bovine growth hormone (rbGH), which in turn was used to stimulate milk production in farm animals. Treatment of dairy cows with rbGH increased production by at least 14% and decreased the amount of feed needed per gallon of milk produced.[47] Based on data from more than 10 years of rbGH studies, the FDA concluded that milk from rbGH-treated cows was safe for human consumption. Recombinant DNA technology has also been applied to produce other proteins important for agriculture and medicine. Subunit vaccines against animal viruses, such as foot and mouth disease virus, are produced by expression of viral coat proteins in bacteria and yeast. The first successful vaccine produced by rDNA technology was the hepatitis B virus (HBV) vaccine. Merck Sharp & Dohme manufactured the HBV vaccine by the rDNA yeast cell method, and HBV vaccine received FDA approval in 1986, and was subsequently used for widespread immunization.

Medical investigators have utilized molecular genetic technology to create innovative gene therapy approaches. Gene therapy is a treatment directed at the gene expression level to replace defective genetic material, or alter the phenotype of target cells for the purpose of preventing or curing a particular disease. The target cells are isolated from the body, grown in culture, genetically manipulated, and then returned to the patient from whom the original cells were removed.

In the past, physicians have treated genetic disorders not by directly altering genes, but by preventing symptomatic conditions. The primary means of preventing complications in individuals with phenylketonuria was dietary restriction, which reduced toxic buildup of the amino acid metabolite, phenylalanine. Since the 1970s, gene therapy has been assessed as a treatment option for cystic fibrosis, muscular dystrophy, adenosine deaminase deficiency, and familial hypercholesterolemia.

The critical step for successful gene therapy is selecting a vector able to serve as a safe and effective gene carrier. An ideal gene vector is a modified virus that can transfer genes to cells but will not replicate or cause disease. Viruses utilized for this purpose include retroviruses and adenoviruses. These viruses have been shown to integrate genes into the host chromosomes without causing disease manifestations. However, random viral vector DNA integration into host chromosomes does. Random vector DNA integration can disrupt host genes, reduce efficiency for integrating selected genes, or increase susceptibility to attack by the host immune system.

Nonviral carriers, such as liposomes, were adapted for therapeutic gene transfer. Liposomes comprise small lipid spheres (lipopleses) and plasmid DNA. Perhaps in the future, investigators will be able to select a particular gene delivery system based on the intended therapeutic goal, alter the level of specific gene expression, or deactivate unwanted integrated genes.[28]

Gene therapy can also be used to target cancer cells; integrated genes would contain the genetic instructions to produce a specific therapeutic protein directed toward malignant cells. One gene therapy strategy involves modifying a patient's cancer cells, e.g., malignant melanoma, with genes encoding for cytokines. A patient's tumor cells are removed; genes to express T-lymphocyte growth factor interleukin-2 (IL-2), or the dendritic cell activator, granulocyte-macrophage colony stimulating factor (GM-CSF), are inserted. The genetically modified tumor cells are infused back into the patient's body, where increased cytokine production results in enhanced immune system activation. The activated immune cells can circulate through the body and attack the tumors.[29]

The promise of effective gene therapy has enormous potential to provide treatment options for incurable diseases and diseases unresponsive to conventional therapy. Possibilities will become more realistic when vectors can more safely and effectively be administered to patients to insert genetic information into specific target cells.

D. Diet Factors and Drug Discovery in Cancer Research

Carcinogenesis is a multiple-step process that involves genetic and environmental factors. Its risk is strongly influenced by individual lifestyle, including dietary choices. The incidence of certain cancer varies geographically and is postulated to be attributable to preferred lifestyles. In Japan, stomach cancer has been the primary cause of cancer for many years. Recent trends, however, show decreasing stomach and uterine cancer rates, and increasing incidences of lung, colon, and breast cancer. These changes may be caused by changes in Japanese dietary habits since World War II. There has been a decrease in intake of dietary fiber and an increased consumption of meat and animal fats in the past 20 years. The increase in colon, breast, ovarian, and prostate cancers is considered to be a result of dietary changes that more closely resemble Western culture. The effect of lifestyle on cancer incidence was markedly demonstrated among immigrants from Asia to North America. Japanese men living in Los Angeles have a combined colon and rectal cancer incidence rate two times that of those living in Miyagi, Japan.

Epidemiological studies have provided supporting evidence that a diet high in saturated fat and low in fiber increased the risk of developing colorectal adenoma. Nitroso compound is considered an initiator of stomach cancer. Quantitative analysis of nitroso-amino acid showed a correlation between gastric cancer mortality rates and urinary nitroso-proline and nitroso-thioproline levels. Dietary preferences in Japan for green and yellow vegetables, tea, and fish, in conjunction with modest animal fat consumption, appear to be associated with lower cancer incidence. The isoflavonoids, daidzein and genistein, found in tofu (soybean curd) could contain factors responsible for preventing colon and estrogen-related cancers.

Colon cancer and adenoma patients are observed to have higher fecal cholesterol metabolites, which include secondary bile acids and neutral metabolites. Enteric flora degrades bile acids to produce hydrolase and 7-alpha-dehydroxylase, which in turn catalyze deconjugation and dehydroxylation, respectively. The enzymatic activities of 7-alpha-dehydroxylase, beta-glucuronidase, nitroreductase, and azoreductase from the fecal microflora in omnivores were found to be higher than in vegetarians. Epidemiologic data support the association between increased fiber consumption and decreased risk for colon cancer. This protective effect may in part be due to the acidic colonic environment created when fiber is degraded into volatile fatty acids, and subsequent dilution of bile acids in the feces.

Japanese men have one of the lowest incidences of prostate cancer in the world. In contrast, prostate cancer in African-American men is approximately 15 times greater than observed in the Japanese population. Prostate cancer mortality rates in the U.S. from 1953 through 1992 increased from approximately 14 to 16 deaths/100,000, whereas the mortality rate in Japan increased from an estimated 1 to 4 deaths/100,000. Prostate cancer is thought to be influenced by hormones; fat may play a role in hormonal etiology. Development of early-stage prostate cancer may be influenced by androgens, particularly dihydrotestosterone, which is formed from testosterone by the 5α-reductase enzyme. Japanese men appear to have low 5α-reductase activity relative to an American population. Differences in 5α-reductase activity may partly explain low prostate cancer rates observed in the Asian population. In addition, a significant fraction of Japanese men developing latent forms of prostate cancer contained inactivating mutations within the androgen receptor gene. However, no such mutations were found in a disease-matched American population. This finding suggests that androgen receptor gene mutations in latent tumors may have a protective effect in Japanese men. A study to evaluate the effect of daily oral α-tocopherol (vitamin E) and β-carotene ingestion on cancer rates among Finnish males showed 34% fewer cases of diagnosed prostate cancer and 16% fewer cases of colorectal cancer in the treatment group.[30,31]

Many kinds of herbal medicines have been used for centuries in Japan and China to improve overall health and treat diseases. A number of phenolic compounds have been identified in herbal medicines and their biological activities extensively studied for possible application to cancer prevention. Screening tests of the phenolic compounds from herbal medicines were carried out to identify compounds with immunostimulating, antioxidative activities and/or antitumor promoting effect.

Russian athletes and cosmonauts use *Eleutherococcus* (Siberian ginseng) as an endurance-enhancing drug. Ginseng and many other herbal medicines contain lignans. (+)-Syringaresinol di-O-β-D-glucoside was isolated as the major component from both *Eleutherococcus* and *Cortex eucommiae*. Lignan has been found to exhibit cyclic AMP phosphodiesterase inhibitory activity, which is linked to the therapeutic effect of antipsychotic, antianxiety, and antihypertensive drugs. It was also observed to have an anti-gastric ulcer effect in restrained, cold-water-stressed rats, and enhanced plasma β-endorphin levels. β-endorphin acts on T-lymphocytes to enhance cell proliferation and natural killer cell activation. Enhanced immune response can provide possible resistance to cancer. Furthermore, (+)-syringaresinol, the aglycone of diglucoside, shows a strong radical-scavenging activity compared with α-tocopherol.[31] Free radicals are implicated in cancer development due to their ability to damage nuclear DNA in the cell and weaken overall immune activity. In a strong antioxidant defense system, the free radical is neutralized before it can damage DNA. Therefore, (+)-syringaresinol di-O-β-glucoside has possible uses as a cancer-preventive drug.

Some compounds isolated from herbal medicines, e.g., mauritianin, a flavonoid from *Herba catharanthi,* arctigenin and trachelogenin, and lignans from *Caulis trachelospermi* are reported to exhibit antitumor-promoting activity.[32] It is hoped that continued studies of herbal medicines can identify effective compounds for future cancer-preventive or therapeutic products.

III. HIGH COSTS OF HEALTH CARE AND DRUG DEVELOPMENT

Advances in medical science and technology undoubtedly contribute to prolonged life expectancy and expected maintenance of good health. Extended life expectancy has created new problems for the current health-care system. The rapid rise of chronic disease conditions is also associated with social and emotional problems. Discounted health insurance and government-subsidized health care have, in fact, stimulated greater utilization of more expensive medical technologies, which has resulted in higher health-care costs and the need for more medical subspecialists. The cost of health care in the U.S. is currently one of the largest expenditures and is expected to account for an even greater share of projected national resources.

In 1940, health-care costs comprised 4% of the GNP, which amounted to an average expense of $30/person.[33] Since then, federal health expenditures have grown at a faster rate than the gross national product (GNP). By 1986, an overall total of $458 billion was spent for health care (10.9% of the GNP) with an average of $1837/person. Thus, projections for the year 2000 included a $5551 per person expenditure, which would account for 15% of the GNP.[34] In the early 1950s, the majority of people in the U.S. paid directly for their own hospitalization expenses; the total health care cost for the country was about $13 billion. By 1976, less than 10% of the population paid directly for their hospitalization, and total health-care costs increased to more than $130 billion. This increase represented a tenfold rise in costs over a 25-year period. Most of the cost increase was due to hospitalization and other services covered by health insurance payments.

During and immediately after World War II, an explosive development of new drugs occurred. Many new therapeutic agents, including antibiotics, steroids, tranquilizers, and anticancer agents, were introduced during this period. However, since the 1960s, there has been a significant decrease in the production rate of new drug substances. During the 1957 to 1959 time period, 168 new drugs were developed and used in the American market, but only 39 drugs were developed during the 1969 to 1971 period, and 40 drugs between 1983 and 1986. Introduction of new drug products continues at this low rate in the U.S. today. In contrast, since 1975, the average number of new drugs (new chemical entities, NCEs) acquired from Japan has exceeded the number acquired from the U.S.[35] Major reasons for this transition are the high costs of new drug development due to stricter regulatory requirements and increased public demand for high-quality products. Much more data and evidence for efficacy and safety are required now than in the 1950s. The time, effort, and money required for new drug development has increased more than 1000% during the past 20 years.

The high cost of drug development has become a pressing issue for the pharmaceutical industry. At present, increased attention has focused on dosage form design to improve the rate and intensity of pharmacological response and the duration of drug action. Many manufacturers have concentrated their research on the development of novel dosage forms rather than the discovery of new drug substances. There has been vigorous competition among smaller pharmaceutical companies to market generic products once a drug substance is no longer under patent protection. Economic, political, sociological, scientific, and technological factors all affect the cost of drug development. The FDA as well as the general public is well aware of the extensive costs of drug evaluation. Those in government, industry, and academia frequently ask, "How much does it cost FDA to evaluate and approve one new drug or biological product?" Consequently, cost-benefit and cost-effectiveness analyses have been conducted on various vaccines, such as pertussis, polio, pneumococcal disease, and hepatitis B.[36–41]

Recently, the Center for Biologics Evaluation and Research, FDA, analyzed the human resource expenditures for licensure of Merck Sharp & Dohme's Haemophilus b conjugate vaccine (PedvaxHIB).[42] The investigational new drug (IND) application for this product was filed on January 30, 1984. The product license application (PLA) was filed on November 17, 1987. The product was licensed on December 20, 1989, which was 2 years and 1 month after the filing of the PLA. The total prelicensing review time was 71 months (IND — 46 months; PLA — 25 months). Estimates were also provided for an additional 17 months' postlicensure experience, ending May 29, 1991. A total of 42 scientists and technical personnel were involved in reviewing documents, and evaluating data and control tests to ensure that the product was effective and safe. Thus, enormous human resources with extraordinary effort were mobilized to evaluate this biological product. The reports on cost-benefit analysis of vaccines show that the immunization represents a remarkably effective use of limited resources and that expenditure of funds on immunization reaps benefits well in excess of that expenditure. For example, the analysis of the benefits and costs of the measles, mumps, and rubella (MMR) vaccine demonstrated savings of $11.90, $6.70, and $7.70, respectively, for every dollar invested. Using a combined MMR vaccine approach, savings increased to $14.40 for every dollar invested.[43] These results indicate that immunization is one of the most cost-effective ways to prevent disease.

IV. DRUG SAFETY AND GLOBAL HEALTH

An adverse drug reaction (ADR) has been defined as any response to a drug that is noxious and unintended and occurs at doses used in humans for prophylaxis, diagnosis, and therapy. In many cases, the FDA approves drugs and biological products under the condition that continuing studies of safety and stability be conducted to investigate rare adverse reactions or long-term effects. Both the FDA and manufacturers closely monitor drugs and biological products postlicensure.

Although development of modern drugs and vaccines is strictly controlled, these products are nevertheless neither perfectly safe nor absolutely effective, even when properly used. Since the manufacturing and sale of drugs are regulated by the government, and most childhood vaccines are mandatory, many people consider that society has an obligation to provide compensation for vaccine-related reactions. Because high universal immunization rates cause the incidence of vaccine-preventable diseases to become a rare occurrence, tolerance for vaccine-related adverse events also lessens.

A higher standard of safety is generally expected of vaccines than drugs because vaccines are largely given to healthy people. Tolerance for adverse reactions in a healthy population is much lower than in a diseased population. The general public shows greater concern for rare adverse events, such as acute encephalopathy after immunization with whole-cell pertussis vaccine, or Guillain-Barre syndrome (GBS) after swine influenzae vaccination, than for frequent toxic side effects from cancer chemotherapy. There is also little attention paid to 30%

of people who experience GI symptoms following receipt of high-dose aspirin.

In recent years, large numbers of lawsuits have been filed against manufacturers to demand injury compensation caused by adverse drug reactions. Rising liability costs are in turn factored into the initial price of the approved product. For example, during the period from 1983 to 1986, the price of diphtheria, tetanus, and pertussis (DTP) combined vaccine in the private sector increased from approximately $0.12/dose to $11.00/dose. Several manufacturers of DTP ceased production and distribution, leaving only one manufacturer (Wyeth–Lederle) to supply vaccine for the entire U.S. This led to a DTP vaccine shortage and the need for abbreviated immunization schedules.[44] In order to alleviate problems of vaccine-related liability, the National Vaccine Injury Act was passed by the U.S. Congress in 1986. Provision for a review process to determine compensation for vaccine-related injuries was established.[45]

Manufacturers are required by law to report all adverse reactions to the FDA. This includes information related to the use of drugs and biologics in professional practice, overdose or withdrawal, and any significant failure in expected pharmacological action. An unexpected adverse reaction is an event that is not described in the labeling for the product. A serious adverse experience is an event occurring at any dose that is fatal or life threatening, that results in disability or congenital anomaly, and requires hospitalization or surgical operation to prevent impairment of physiological function or permanent disability.

The FDA considers adverse event reporting essential to provide continued assurance of safety and effectiveness of licensed drugs, biologics, and medical devices. Even the most extensive animal studies and clinical trials cannot detect all possible adverse reactions. Clinical trials using a few thousand people over a period of months or years may not always identify a rare adverse event. Oral polio vaccine-associated paralytic polio, which occurs at a rate of 1 in 10,000 vaccinated persons, was more accurately estimated during postmarketing surveillance. Moreover, drugs and biologics are tested in a limited number of high-risk populations, e.g., the elderly and young children, and rarely in pregnant women. Since it is not possible to assess all combinations of concomitant medications, persons simultaneously taking multiple drugs may experience drug interactions or incompatibilities not detected during prelicensure animal and clinical studies.

Because rare adverse reactions, reactions with delayed onset, or reactions in subpopulations may not be detected before drugs or biologics are licensed, postmarketing evaluation of drug and vaccine safety is important. In the past, this evaluation has relied on passive surveillance and epidemiological studies. More recently, Phase IV trials and pre-established large-linked databases (LLDBs) have been added to improve capabilities to study rare risks possibly associated with drug therapies and immunizations. Postmarketing surveillance systems may also detect potential manufacturing and lot-specific variations in a timely manner.

Postmarketing observational study results are confounded by participant bias. Individuals who are extremely health conscious or chronically suffer from undiagnosed medical conditions are more likely to enroll in a clinical study. Passive surveillance or spontaneous reporting systems (SRS) have traditionally been used for postmarketing vaccine safety monitoring due to the relatively low cost incurred. In many countries, adverse event reporting is linked to the agency that purchases vaccines for the public sector. In the U.S., a large proportion of vaccines are purchased by the Centers for Disease Control and Prevention (CDC). This agency purchases more than half of the childhood vaccines used in the U.S. In many developing countries, the Ministry of Health, in conjunction with the World Health Organization's Expanded Programme on Immunization (EPI), administers almost all childhood vaccines. Any adverse events thought to be vaccine related are first reported to the organization that administered the vaccine. Since both the CDC and FDA have a vested interest in vaccine safety, the vaccine adverse event reporting system has become a joint collaborative effort.

The FDA has established an adverse event reporting system called MEDWatch, the FDA Medical Products Reporting Program. Under this system, adverse drug reactions, drug quality problems, device quality problems, and adverse reactions due to medical devices have been combined into a single reporting form (FDA Form 3500A) for health professionals. Physicians and health-care personnel should file a report whenever a drug or biological product is suspected to have caused a serious adverse event. Manufacturers should report all adverse events, both serious and unexpected, to the FDA within 15 days of becoming aware of the event.

Enactment of the National Childhood Vaccine Injury Act also mandated physicians and other health-care personnel to keep permanent immunization records and voluntarily report specific vaccine-induced adverse events. A vaccine injury table was established to specify a timeframe within which a reportable event could occur following immunization. Adverse events associated with vaccines are reported through the Vaccine Adverse Event Reporting System (VAERS), which is a joint program sponsored by the FDA and the CDC. Since its inception in late 1990, approximately 10,000 VAERS reports have been received annually, of which 20% have been categorized as serious adverse events. VAERS is useful for detecting initial signals of unrecognized adverse reactions following vaccination. It is the only surveillance system with a database encompassing the entire U.S. population. It is, therefore, the major means to detect possible new, unusual, or rare adverse events. To further promote international agreement, adverse experience reports derived from foreign countries may be submitted on a form provided by the Council for International Organizations of Medical Sciences (CIOMS).

The 20th century brought forth a global network of pharmaceutical companies with an extraordinary research and new drug development capability. This biopharmaceutical network, however, has focused primarily on the health problems of affluent nations. Primary goals depend on large profit margins from successfully developed drugs and biologic products. Inflated prices widened the gap for global access to adequate health care. The price gap between rich and poor countries arises from differing national priorities and government policy, as well as from tremendous financial differences in the ability to pay for newly approved products. As a result, multiple initiatives were created to address the growing global drug gap problem.

The World Health Organization (WHO) estimates that one third of the world's population does not have access to essential drugs, which include 302 active ingredients, e.g., ibuprofen, mebendazole, and ampicillin. This organization aids a country's capacity to purchase necessary drugs through drug procurement. The United Nations Children's Fund (UNICEF) was also established as a procurement service, which offers to purchase essential drugs on behalf of developing countries at discounted prices.

On a national level, efforts to optimize domestic production capacity should also be initiated to establish a sound distribution system and means to maintain an adequate supply. Constructive solutions are needed to perpetuate incentives for research and drug development, and to reduce the inequities of access to these products.

In 1990, more than 4 billion people, which constitutes over 80% of the world's population, lived in developing countries. In some areas, birth rates are as high as 42 per 1000 population, and the infant mortality rate (IMR) is approximately 12 per 1000 population. The annual population growth, therefore, is 3%. The population patterns in developing countries are comparatively young; the median age is often in the upper teens. In 1990, the overall IMR in low-income countries other than China and India was about 92 deaths per 1000 live births. The IMR per 1000 live births in Nepal, Sierra Leone, Malawi, and Mali was 121, 147, 149 and 166, respectively.[46] In some geographic regions, the IMR may be even higher. In contrast, the IMR in Japan is 6 to 7 deaths per 1000 live births. In the U.S., the IMR remains approximately 10 per 1000 live births. National immunization programs in developing countries focus primarily on childhood vaccines as an important means to prevent infant mortality. Every year, approximately 14 or 15 million children in these countries, who are younger than 5 years old, die; approximately 40,000 children die each day. Many deaths are associated with co-morbid conditions. Perhaps 60% of deaths are in part due to malnutrition; 80% are associated with diarrhea. Acute respiratory infection caused by *Streptococcus pneumoniae, Haemophilus influenzae,* pertussis, measles, and malaria is also a prevailing factor. Many surviving children are left with permanent sequelae. Infection in early life may have serious long-term consequences. The most obvious social benefits from childhood immunization come from increased individual survival to reproductive age. Vaccines that prevent such respiratory disease and hepatic cancer in adulthood are also an important public health initiative. Several principles are considered when a manufacturer develops a vaccine. In contrast to drugs, which are distributed to a broad target population and used repeatedly, a childhood vaccine is given one to five times over the entire human life span. Although a vaccine is given a limited number of times, the target population could potentially involve the entire birth cohort. Not all vaccines, however, are indicated for universal use. Vaccines for prevention of rare diseases, such as Q fever, Japanese encephalitis, or rabies, although safe and effective, have limited or no market in most countries. Despite past records of global public health achievements such as successful introduction of inactivated polio vaccine in 1954, the arrival of live polio and measles vaccines in the succeeding decade, and efforts to reduce the threat of liability through injury compensation, manufacture of vaccines declined steadily through the 1970s to the middle of the 1980s.

From the late 1980s, research and development on vaccines were revived because the pharmaceutical industry realized that new bio-technologies could improve existing vaccines and contribute to the development of newer, more effective vaccines. Equally important were the efforts of national and global organizations to promote "Health for All by the Year 2000" — a goal for all people to attain to a level of health that would permit them to lead socially and economically productive lives.

The WHO plays a central role in immunization programs, especially for developing nations, by funding and facilitating collaboration toward global health initiatives. Before the Expanded Programme on Immunization (EPI) was launched by WHO in 1974, there were very few means to establish an infrastructure to support universal immunization in the poorest countries. The EPI, developed in close collaboration with UNICEF, provides childhood vaccines for six target diseases. Vaccine to prevent diseases caused by diphtheria, pertussis, tetanus, measles, polio, and tuberculosis were provided, as well as much of the supplies and equipment needed for vaccine administration. The EPI established intermediate targets of 80% by 1990 and 90% by 2000, with an eventual goal of 100% universal immunization coverage. In April 1992, global immunization coverage had reached 88% for BCG, 82% for DTP, 84% for a third dose of polio vaccine, and 80% for measles vaccine during the first year of life. The EPI subsequently made great efforts to improve cold chain technology and vaccine thermostability, which would benefit vaccine administration in remote regions of tropical countries.

The International Vaccine Institute (IVI) was established in the early 1990s as part of the Children's Vaccine Initiative (CVI), which is sponsored by the World Bank, WHO, UNICEF, and the Rockefeller Foundation, to develop new vaccines and upgrade existing vaccines for developing countries. Major goals and objectives of the IVI include:

- To conduct research activities to develop new vaccines and improve the quality of existing vaccines
- To assist in regional vaccine production and quality control and regulation of vaccines
- To coordinate multisite clinical trials and field testing of new vaccines
- To provide personnel and financial resources for CVI programs

Seoul was selected as the site for IVI. The Korean government is committed to supporting this international organization on vaccine research and development.

Many international organizations, including the Organization for Economic Cooperation and Development (OECD), the European Community (EC), and the Japan International Cooperation Agency (JICA), are heavily involved in supporting biomedical research, vaccine development, and the promotion of global health. Up to the present time, vaccine development has exclusively focused on preventing childhood diseases. However, new applications of immunization have expanded the scope of vaccine development to include prevention of disease in an older population. Vaccines may be used in adults and the elderly for control of chronic diseases. For example, hepatitis B virus vaccine is utilized in large part to reduce the incidence of hepatic carcinoma. A vaccine consisting of Epstein-Barr virus (EBV) surface glycoprotein, gp340, has been produced in the U.K. and is intended to prevent nasopharyngeal carcinoma. A vaccine against *Helicobacter pylori* is intended to prevent gastric cancer. Vaccines may eventually be developed against cardiovascular and other degenerative diseases such as Alzheimer's disease.

It is hoped that ultimately these scientific endeavors will succeed through the collaborations among scientists, pharmaceutical industry, regulatory agencies, and the enthusiasm of the global community.

V. SCIENTIFIC ADVANCES TO REVOLUTIONIZE MODERN MEDICINE

As we enter the 21st century, we are approaching a historic transition in medicine and pharmaceutical sciences. A few years ago, only little pieces of the genetic information of life, the genomes, were understood in detail. After dramatic advances in molecular genetics and biotechnology, the complete sequence of the human genome has become available. Information processing on computers and biomedical science are crucial in this progress and epic transition. The potential impact on biomedicine, health care, and quality of life is expected to be enormous.

A. Gene Technology and Stem Cells for Medical Therapeutics

In 1995, two lambs were born from a surrogate mother that received genetic material from cultured embryonic cells. The successful cloning proved that even though the cultured cells are partially differentiated, they can be genetically reprogrammed to function like those in an early embryo. Most biomedical investigators had believed that this was impossible. Later, the cultured cells taken from a 26-day-old fetus and from a mature ewe were cloned to animals. In February 1997, the ewe's cells produced Dolly, the first mammal to be cloned from an adult. The possibility to create clones from tissue culture cells brought forth alternative ways to develop beneficial medical therapeutic drugs, practical benefits in animal husbandry, and a more in-depth understanding of the mechanisms contributing to cell development.

Cloning is based on nuclear transfer that involves the use of two cells. The recipient cell is an unfertilized egg taken from an animal soon after ovulation. The donor cell is the one to be copied. During the cloning process, chromosomes from the recipient egg are gently removed by a micropipette. Then, the donor cell with an intact nucleus is fused with the recipient egg. When implanted into a surrogate mother, the fused cells continue to develop similarly to a normal embryo. The cloning of Dolly from the mammary-derived culture, and cloning of other lambs from the cultured fibroblasts, showed that the cloned offspring looked like the sheep that donated the nucleus, rather than like their surrogate mothers. Genetic tests prove that Dolly is indeed a clone of an adult.

Investigators then inserted the gene for human factor IX, a blood-clotting protein used to treat hemophilia, into sheep. Also, an antibiotic-resistance gene was transferred to the donor cells along with the factor IX gene, so a high dose of the antibiotic neomycin added to cultured cells selected only those that contained the transferred gene. In 1997, the first transgenic sheep was produced by this method. The transgenic animals secreted the human protein in their milk.

Cloning has many other practical applications. One is the supply of genetically modified animal organs that are suitable for human transplantation. At present, thousands of patients die before a replacement heart, liver, or kidney becomes available. A normal animal organ would be rapidly destroyed by the body's own immune system, a reaction which is triggered by an alpha-galactosyl transferase enzyme, when the organ is transplanted into a human. Thus, animal organs have been genetically altered so that they no longer contain this enzyme and are better tolerated in the host. Cloning technology provides a means to quickly produce large animal models that mimic human diseases, such as cystic fibrosis. These techniques are also useful in evaluating cell-based therapies for genetic disorders such as muscular dystrophy, diabetes, and Parkinson's disease. There is currently no fully effective treatment for these illnesses.

One of the most important biomedical research initiatives involves the production of universal human donor cells. A difficult challenge is to create cells for transplantation that are not seen as foreign by the recipient immune system. Scientists are investigating the possibility of using undifferentiated embryonic stem cells to repair or replace tissue damaged by disease. Stem cells matched to a patient can be made by using nuclear transfer cloning techniques; this is a technique in which one of the patient's cells serves as the donor and a human egg serves as the recipient. The resulting embryo develops until it is possible to separate and culture stem cells from it. When stem cells divide, some of the progeny differentiate and mature into cells of specific types. Other progeny remain as stem cells. Thus, intestinal stem cells continually regenerate the lining of the intestine, and hematopoietic stem cells produce the cells found in blood. The stem cells enable our bodies to repair diseased tissues, and perhaps can be used to treat AIDS, muscular dystrophy, and Parkinson's disease.

The stem cells can be manipulated to differentiate into specific cells and tissues. Investigators have shown that treating mouse embryonic stem cells with a vitamin A derivative, retinoic acid, stimulated them to produce neurons. Specific growth factors stimulated cells derived from embryonic stem cells to produce the complete range of cells found in blood. Embryonic stem cells could even generate useful tissues without special treatment. Spontaneous differentiation of stem cells was observed to form cardiomyocytes of greater than 99% purity.

B. Cancer and Chronic Diseases in an Aging Society

Since the beginning of the 20th century, the size of the elderly population in the U.S. has been steadily increasing. At present, people 65 years of age and older are expected to live an average of an additional 16 years. Cancer is becoming a larger health problem, and the medicines used as treatments have limitations. In the U.S., cancer is the second leading cause of death and is expected to become the leading cause in the near future. The medical treatment of cancer still has many pitfalls. The mainstay of cancer treatment, surgery and radiation, is generally only effective if the cancer is found at an early and localized stage. When the disease has progressed to an advanced metastatic stage, these therapies are less successful. In many cases, the chemotherapies are effective only for a short period.

The development of new drugs and biologic products for cancer therapy involves several critical issues. Ideal therapies would include targeted and lasting antitumor activity, low toxicities, and avoidance of drug resistance caused by the genomic instability of tumors. Biomedical research discoveries based on disease mechanisms often lead to the most direct pharmaceutical approaches to counter the disease. During the past 20 years, there has been a basic change in the way target identification in cancer is approached. Progress in molecular genetics now allows scientists to identify genes that become deranged in cancer. At first, there were just a few cancer genes such as *src, abl,* and *ras.* At present, many genes are known to affect tumorigenesis and tumor growth. Various areas of signal transduction, cell-cycle regulation, apoptosis, telomere biology, and angiogenesis are studied extensively to select potential therapeutic molecular targets against tumor cells. These molecular targets include EGF, epidermal growth factor receptor; ER, estrogen receptor; Ftase, farnesyltransferase; and PKC, protein kinase C. The choice of target is often based on the underlying gene mutation. Overexpression of specific gene products, such as HER-2, epidermal growth factor, and insulin-like growth factor receptor, has been considered as a causative factor in cancers. In addition, a normal gene product may be correlated with cancer progression. Elevated telomerase activity is observed in all human cancers, and increased serum vascular endothelial growth factor (VEGF) has been found to correlate with decreased survival rates in patients with breast, ovarian, lung, gastric, and colon cancer. These findings indicate that the telomerase enzyme and the KDR receptor of VEGF are good targets for cancer drug development. Some of the most exciting results are reported with agents directed against tyrosine kinase, either as therapeutic antibodies or as small-molecule kinase inhibitors. Many molecular mechanisms have been examined as new targets for drug development in the hope that they will have more effective antitumor activity.[50]

The hard medical reality is that prostate cancer kills. This disease is the second leading cause of cancer death in men in the U.S. and results in more than 32,000 deaths each year. It is especially prevalent in men older than 65 years of age. For most men, neither computed tomography (CT) scans nor standard ultrasound procedures can provide a clear picture of a tumor or its spread beyond the prostate gland. Recently, an ultrasound technique has shown promise in applying a signal-processing technology known as spectrum analysis. Sound waves are bounced off the prostate and analyzed as sound echoes. Then, sophisticated computer programming translates the data into a three-dimensional view of the gland, complete with color to highlight the tumor. New approaches for prostate cancer imaging by magnetic resonance (MRI) are also under study. MRI devices emit magnetic fields around a patient to produce cross-sectional images of the body. When a patient has a small emitter of electromagnetic waves inserted into his rectum, the resulting views can show whether, and how far, the tumor has grown past the prostate gland. Magnetic resonance spectroscopy, which measures metabolic activity in a viewed area, may further help distinguish between normal and cancerous tissue.[51,52]

The goal of surgery for the prostate is threefold: to remove cancer within the prostate; to preserve urinary control following surgery; and to preserve erectile function. Prior to the advent of laparoscopic surgery, the typical incision for open radical prostatectomy would be 8 inches. Recent advances in surgery techniques can further extend survival time and improve the quality of life for many prostate cancer patients. Now, with a groundbreaking new technique called laparoscopic prostatectomy, improved surgical outcome and greater quality of life is possible. This revolutionary approach uses a video camera to magnify the operative field twelvefold. Better operative precision leads to greater preservation of vital anatomic structures. Careful attention is paid to avoiding delicate nerves adjacent to the cancer. The best news of all is that this technique offers the advantage of smaller scars, less pain medication, less blood loss, and quicker return to normal life.

Because many human diseases are caused by heredity and central nervous system disorders, it is exciting to see how biomedical research has contributed to the early detection, prevention, and treatment of geriatric conditions such as Alzheimer's disease, depression, and Parkinson's disease. The dramatic rise in life expectancy has enabled many of us to reach the age at which degenerative chromic disorders, such as Alzheimer's disease and stroke, become common. Approximately 15% of people who live to the age of 65 will develop some form of dementia; by age 85, the proportion increases to at least 35%. Of all the dementias, Alzheimer's disease is the most common. Understanding the accumulation of β-amyloid protein plaques that occur in the brain provides significant clues about disease mechanisms. Deposits of amyloid protein gather in the spaces between nerve cells. Amyloid plaques are usually accompanied by reactive inflammatory cells called microglia, which are part of the brain's immune system trying to degrade and remove damaged neurons. Such plaques are present in most elderly people. Their extensive presence, however, in the hippocampus and the cerebral cortex is specific to Alzheimer's patients. The amyloid protein is a small fragment, made up of either 40 or 42 amino acids. Identification of the β-amyloid peptide was made possible by sequencing the 695-amino acid protein referred to as the β-amyloid precursor protein (βAPP). The βAPP gene is located on chromosome 21. People with Down's syndrome, who have three rather than two copies of chromosome 21, invariably display some features of Alzheimer's by the age of 40. These findings suggest that the amyloid protein is involved in the onset of Alzheimer's disease, and the βAPP gene may be the site of mutations.

In the course of Alzheimer's disease βAPP is processed in one of two ways. The protein is first cleaved by the alpha-secretase and gamma-secretase enzymes. The resulting product is a harmless peptide fragment called p3. The second way in which βAPP is cleaved involves another two-step process. First, the protein is cleaved by a beta-secretase to form a C99-βAPP fragment. This fragment is then cleaved by gamma-secretase to form the β-amyloid peptide. The peptide may act in several ways. First, it disrupts calcium regulation, which can lead to cell death. Second, it damages mitochondria, causing the release of free oxygen radicals, which then damage proteins, lipids, and DNA. Third, it causes neuronal injury and release of cellular compounds. An inflammatory response may occur, which creates a cycle of escalating damage.

New treatments for Alzheimer's focus on blocking the ability of either the beta- or gamma-secretase enzyme to cleave APP, thus preventing β-amyloid peptide formation. Other alternative approaches include antioxidants, such as glycoaminoglycans, which can break down β-amyloid aggregates. Attempts have also been made to develop a therapeutic vaccine to neutralize the activity of β-amyloid peptide.[53] Whatever the future holds, it is increasingly likely that, in the years to come, more effective products and treatments will be generated.

C. New Efforts in Countering Bioterrorism

September 11, 2001, marked the beginning of a dark autumn. From the moment two hijacked airplanes crashed into the World Trade Center towers, an attack that killed thousands of people, biomedical scientists realized the imminent threat of bioterrorism. The attack showed that these terrorists were sophisticated, organized, and, perhaps, capable of producing biologic weapons of mass destruction. They were able and willing to destroy large numbers of people. Thus, on October 4, 2001, when cases of anthrax disease were identified in an office building in Florida, in an NBC employee in New York, among staff in the U.S. Senate majority leader's office, and in postal workers in Washington, D.C., the suspected existence of biological weapons was confirmed. By December 5, 2001, a total of 22 cases of anthrax had been identified; 11 were confirmed as inhalational anthrax and 11 were cutaneous.[54]

In 1995, the year that sarin gas attacks in the Tokyo subway killed 12 and injured thousands, U.S. President Bill Clinton made counter-terrorism a top priority. Federal resources were allocated to strengthen counter-terrorism initiatives. In fiscal year 1998, the Department of Health and Human Services (HHS) budget for countering bioterrorism was about $2 million. It has since grown to $175 million. Budget allocations for the years 2002/2003 currently amount to $1.7 billion.

According to a government study, a mere 100 kg of anthrax released from an airplane above a metropolitan area could spread an invisible, odorless cloud of spores that could kill 130,000 to 3 million people. Anthrax is a particularly difficult challenge because so little is known about it. Inhalation anthrax has been associated with farmers who have inhaled its spores from contaminated animal hides, wool, and fur. There were only 18 identified cases of inhalation anthrax in the U.S. in the 20th century, and most of those occurred before the age of antibiotics. More information about inhalation anthrax was obtained from an accidental anthrax release at a Russian bioweapons facility in 1979. A germ warfare facility in Sverdlovsk, Russia, accidentally released an aerosol of the pathogen and killed at least 70 people. The average incubation period for onset of inhalation anthrax is 11 days after exposure. In preparation for future anthrax attacks, large stockpiles of antibiotics would have to be kept on hand for immediate use. Anticipated supply would need to account for exposure involving millions of people, and a 60-day treatment for each individual exposure.

There is little experience thus far involving deliberate release of biological agents. However, events of recent years have indicated the increasing possibility of such incidents, particularly terrorist incidents aimed at the civilian population. In addition to anthrax, concerns about deliberate use of disease agents is now focused on smallpox, bubonic plague, tularemia, viral hemorrhagic fevers, and botulism. While there are vaccines or treatments available for these diseases, they do not exist in massive stockpiles. Smallpox, while eradicated as a naturally occurring disease, could cause a chain reaction of person-to-person infection if ever released in a terrorist attack.

In preparing for possible bioterrorist incidents, health-care agencies face new challenges. Unlike explosives or chemical releases, a bioterrorist attack will not be evident until symptoms appear days or weeks later. A strong public health network is needed to coordinate early reports and implement contingency plans. The medical and health-care community need an improved network of infectious disease surveillance, including a rapid reporting system, effective diagnostic techniques and laboratory facilities, and expanded training of health-care personnel.

To better detect and respond to a wide range of infectious disease threats and possible bioterrorist incidents, the CDC is planning to intensify efforts to upgrade the nation's public health laboratory and epidemiological survey capability. The agency will also help expand training and communication capacities for state and local health agencies. The National Pharmaceutical Stockpile Program will be established to maintain a national repository of life-saving pharmaceuticals in the event of a bioterrorist attack. The HHS will expand support for research related to possible bioterrorism agents. The National Institutes of Health (NIH) will emphasize research to determine genomic sequence information of potential bioterrorism agents such as anthrax, tularemia, and plague. Genomic and other biomedical research will help in developing rapid diagnostic methods, new or improved antibacterial and antiviral therapies, and new vaccines.[55,56]

The U.S. anthrax vaccine, an inactivated cell-free product, was licensed in 1970 and is produced by BioPort Corp., Lansing, MI (formerly called the Michigan Biologic Products Institute). The vaccine is approved as a six-dose series for U.S. military active- and reserve-duty personnel. The vaccine is prepared from the cell-free filtrate of a noncapsulated attenuated strain of *Bacillus anthracis*. A similar vaccine has been reported efficacious against cutaneous anthrax. As of March 1999, approximately 590,000 doses of anthrax vaccine had been given to U.S. armed forces. There were no confirmed serious adverse events related to vaccination. Current vaccine supplies are limited, and it will take years before production levels are such that quantities sufficient for civilian use can be produced. Select vaccination of medical personnel who would respond first to a suspected case of bioterrorism is also being considered. Ciprofloxacin or other fluoroquinolone therapy is recommended in adults with inhalational anthrax infection.

Smallpox was eradicated in 1980. The only known remaining samples of the virus are maintained in the U.S. CDC and at the State Research Center of Virology and Biotechnology in Novosibirsk, Siberia. After the Soviet Union collapsed, terrorists were suspected of obtaining smallpox from Novosibirsk. The U.S. currently has 15 million doses of aging smallpox vaccine, which is not enough to provide adequate military and civilian protection. Therefore, in 1997, an arrangement was made with DynPort Vaccine Co., a British–U.S. joint venture based in Frederick, MD, to make 300,000 doses of a new smallpox vaccine for the military. Investigators at the U.S. Army Medical Research Institute of Infectious Diseases (USAMRIID), the leading military lab, tried to grow vaccinia in tissue culture for greater purity and to develop a more effective vaccine. DynPort started working on the tissue-grown vaccinia project in 1998. In September 2000, CDC awarded a 20-year, $343-million contract to Ora Vax, a Cambridge, MA, biotech company; the price was estimated at $1.38 per dose. Both DynPort and Ora Vax (which later changed its name to Acambis) subcontracted responsibilities to another company, BioReliance of Rockville, MD. After September 2001, at CDC's request Acambis accelerated its production schedule in order to be finished by the summer of 2002.

In the meantime, scientists at the National Institute of Allergy and Infectious Diseases (NIAID), NIH, are conducting studies to assess the immunogenicity of diluted existing supplies of smallpox vaccine. NIAID is also helping the CDC with the clinical testing needed for licensure of the new Acambis vaccine.[57] All efforts are being made to ensure that adequate smallpox vaccine is available for both the military and civilian populations within several days if infection occurs in the future.

During the 20th century, basic research in biomedicine and pharmaceutical sciences significantly contributed to the development of new drugs and biologic products. In addition, advances in biotechnology led to the identification of many molecules important in disease processes. These new technology and biological products raised important new regulatory challenges. Recombinant DNA-derived therapeutics licensed in recent years have revolutionized the treatment of heart disease, cancer, serious infections, arthritis, anemia, hemophilia, multiple sclerosis, and many other diseases.

As we enter the 21st century, more biologic products have been licensed. Examples of these products include new polysaccharide and conjugate vaccines for Haemophilus b, pneumococcus, and meningococcus; combination vaccines such as diphtheria, tetanus, and acellular pertussis; and other vaccines such as typhoid, rabies, hepatitis B and A virus, and chickenpox. New biological products also include the first HIV test system for which blood samples may be collected at home; a device that concentrates adult blood stem cells from bone marrow; and Rh0 (D) Immune Globulin Intravenous, the first human blood product approved for both intravenous and intramuscular use.

This century will be very exciting and challenging. There will be an explosion of new drugs and biologics that, until recently, were only the dreams and aspirations of investigators in research laboratories. In this century, effective AIDS and cancer vaccines are anticipated, as well as safer blood supply and tissue products. We will have new and more effective treatments for Alzheimer's and other chronic diseases.

Advances in proteomics and genomics research will produce individualized medicines that have practical therapeutic benefits and fewer adverse reactions. We welcome the new era of biomedicine and look forward to continuing progress to fulfill dreams of better health and quality of life.

REFERENCES

1. Public Health Service, Healthy people: the surgeon general's report on health promotion and disease prevention, Health and Human Services, U.S. Government Printing Office, Washington, D.C., 1982.
2. Edelman, C.L. and Mandle, C.L., Health defined: promotion and specific protection, in *Health Promotion throughout the Lifespan,* 2nd ed., The C.V. Mosby Company, St. Louis, MO, 1990, 3–15.
3. Snader, T.C., Long-term care facilities, in *Remington's Pharmaceutical Sciences,* 18th ed., Gennaro, A.R. (Ed.), Mark Printing Company, Easton, PA, 1990, 1758–1772.
4. Lee, C.J., Lee, L.H., and Koizumi, K., Polysaccharide vaccines for prevention of encapsulated bacterial infections: part I, *Infect. Med.,* 19(3):127–133, 2002.
5. Lee, C.J., Lee, L.H., and Koizumi, K., Polysaccharide vaccines for prevention of encapsulated bacterial infections: part II, *Infect. Med.,* 19(4):179–182, 2002.
6. Lee, L.H., Lee, C.J., and Frasch, C.E., Development and evaluation of pneumococcal conjugate vaccines: clinical trials and control test, *Crit. Rev. Microbiol.,* 28(1):27–41, 2002.
7. Gurunathan, S., Klinman, D.M., and Seder, R.A., DNA vaccines: immunology, application, and optimization, *Annu. Rev. Immunol.,* 18:927–974, 2000.
8. Weiner D.B. and Kennedy, R.C., Genetic vaccines, *Sci. Am.,* July 1999, 50–57.
9. Tuteja, R., DNA vaccines: a ray of hope, *Crit. Rev. Biochem. Mol. Biol.,* 34(1):1–24, 1999.
10. Seder, R.A. and Gurunathan, S., DNA vaccines — designer vaccines for the 21st century, *N. Engl. J. Med.,* 341;277–278, 1999.
11. Martin, T., Parker, S.E., Hedstrom, R. et al., Plasmic DNA malaria vaccine: the potential for genomic integration after intramuscular injection, *Hum. Gene Ther.,* 10:759–768, 1999.
12. Mor, G., Singla, M., Steinberg, A.D. et al., Do DNA vaccines induce autoimmune disease? *Hum. Gene Ther.,* 8:293–300, 1997.
13. Mor, G., Yamshchikov, G., Sedegah, M. et. al., Induction of neonatal tolerance by plasmid DNA vaccination of mice, *J. Clin. Invest.,* 98:2700–2705, 1996.
14. Ichino, M., Mor, G., Conover, J. et al., Factors associated with the development 1of neonatal tolerance after the administration of a plasmid DNA vaccine, *J. Immunol.,* 162:3814–3818, 1999.
15. Langridge, W.H. Edible vaccines, *Sci. Am.,* September 2000, 66–71,
16. Arntzen, C.J. and Mason, H.S., Oral vaccine production in the edible tissues of transgenic plants, in *New Generation Vaccines,* 2nd ed., revised and expanded, Levine, M.M., Woodrow, G.C., Kaper, J.B., and Cobon, G.S. (Eds.), Marcel Dekker, New York, 1977, 263–277.

17. Mason, H.S., Tacket, C.O., Richter, L.J. et al., Subunit vaccines produced and delivered in transgenic plants as "edible vaccines," *Rev. Immunol.,* 149:71–74, 1998.

17a. Haq, T.A., Mason, H.S., Clements, J.D., and Arntzen, C.J., Production of an orally immunogenic bacterial protein in transgenic plants: proof of concept of edible vaccine, *Science,* 268:714–716, 1995.

17b. Mason, H.S., Ball, J., Shi, J.J. et al., Expression of Norwalk virus capsid protein in transgenic tobacco and potato and its oral immunogenicity, *Proc. Natl. Acad. Sci. USA,* 93:5335–5340, 1996.

18. Eisenberg, D.M., Davis, R.B., Ettner, S.L. et al., Trends in alternative medicine uses in the United States, 1990–1997. Results of a follow-up national survey, *JAMA,* 20:1569–1575, 1998.

19. Bannerman, R., Burton, J., and Chen, W.C. (Eds.), *Traditional Medicine and Health Care Coverage,* World Health Organization, Geneva, Switzerland, 1983.

19a. Lee, K.H., Wang, H.K., Itokawa, H. et al., Current perspectives on Chinese medicines and dietary supplements in China, Japan, and the United States, *J. Food Drug Anal.,* 8(4):219–228, 2000.

20. Hosoya, E., Scientific reevaluation of Kampo prescriptions using modern technology, in *Recent Advances in the Pharmacology of Kampo Medicines,* Hosoya, E. and Yamamura, Y. (Eds.), Excerpta Medica, Tokyo, 1988, 17–29.

21. Kobashi, K., Glycosides are natural prodrugs — evidence using germ-free and gnotobiotic rats associated with a human intestinal bacterium, *J. Trad. Med.,* 15:1–13, 1998.

22. Yamada, H., The role of bioactive polysaccharides in Kampo medicines, in *Pharmacological Research on Traditional Herbal Medicines,* Watanabe, H. and Shibuya, T. (Eds.), Harwood Academic Publishers, Amsterdam, The Netherlands, 2000, 179–198.

23. Lee, C.J., Immunomodulating polysaccharides in plant medicine, in *Managing Biotechnology in Drug Development,* Lee, C.J. (Ed.), CRC Press, Boca Raton, FL, 1966, 120–123.

24. Lee, C.J., Koizumi, K., Koizumi, M., and Aburada, M., Immunomodulating effects of polysaccharides isolated from herbal products, *J. Trad. Med.,* 16:175–182, 1999.

24a. Wetzel, M.S., Kaptchuk, T.J., Haramati, A. et al., Complementary and alternative medical therapies: implication for medical education, *Ann. Intern. Med.,* 138:191–196, 2003.

25. Eisenberg, D.M., Davis, R.B., Ettner, S.L. et al., Trends in alternative medicine use in the United States, 1990–1997, *JAMA,* 280 (18):1569–1609, 1998.

26. Jonas, W.B., Alternative medicine — learning from the past, examine the present, advancing to the future, *JAMA,* 280(18):1616–1618, 1998.

27. Fontanarosa, P.B. and Lundberg, G.D., Alternative medicine meets science, *JAMA,* 280(18):1618–1619, 1998.

28. Brenner, M.K., Human somatic gene therapy: progress and problems, *J. Inter. Med.,* 237:229–239, 1995.

29. Blaese, M., Gene therapy for cancer, *Sci. Am.,* June p. 111–120, 1997.

30. Watanabe, S., Kimira, M., and Sobue, T., Diet and cancer: epidemiological approaches, in *Food Factors for Cancer Prevention,* Ohigashi, H., Osawa, T., Terao, J. et al. (Eds.), Springer-Verlag, Tokyo, 1997, 3–8.

31. Greenwald, P., Diet and cancer prevention in the United States, in *Food Factors for Cancer Prevention*, Ohigashi, H., Osawa, T., Terao, J. et al. (Eds.), Springer-Verlag, Tokyo, 1997, 30–35.

32. Nishibe, S., Bioactive phenolic compounds for cancer prevention from herbal medicines, in *Food Factors for Cancer Prevention*, Ohigashi, H., Osawa, T., Terao, J. et al. (Eds.), Springer-Verlag, Tokyo, 1997, 276–279.

33. Waldo, D.R., Levit, K.R., and Lazenby, H., National health expenditures, 1985, *Health Care Financing Rev.*, 8:1, 1986.

34. Pearson, C., National health expenditures 1986–2000, *Health Care Financing Rev.*, 8(4):1, 1987.

35. DiMasi, J.A., Bryant, N.R., and Lasagna, L., New drug development in the United States from 1963 to 1990, *Clin. Pharmacol. Therap.*, 50:471–486, 1991.

36. Koplan, J.P., Schoenbaum, S.C., Weinstein, M.C., and Fraser, D.W., Pertussis vaccine — an analysis of benefits, risks and costs, *N. Engl. J. Med.*, 301(17):906–911, 1979.

37. Hinman, A.R. and Koplan, J.P., Pertussis and pertussis vaccine — reanalysis of benefits, risks and costs, *JAMA*, 251(23):3109–3113, 1984.

38. Weisbrod, B., Cost and benefits of medical research: a case study of poliomyelitis, *J. Polit. Econ.*, 79:527–544, 1971.

39. Office of Technology Assessment, Update of federal activities regarding the use of pneumococcal vaccine, U.S. Government Printing Office, Washington, D.C., May, 1984.

40. Sisk, J.E. and Riegelman, R.K., Cost effectiveness of vaccination against pneumococcal pneumonia: an update, *Ann. Int. Med.*, 104:79–86, 1986.

41. Kirkman-Liff, B. and Dandoy, S., Cost of hepatitis B prevention in hospital employees: post-exposure prophylaxis, *Infect. Cont.*, 5(8):385–389, 1984.

42. Center for Biologics Evaluation and Research, Human resource expenditures for licensure of MSD's Haemophilus b conjugate vaccine, Food and Drug Administration, Rockville, MD, December 1991.

43. White, C.C., Koplan, J.P., and Orenstein, W.A., Benefits, risks and costs of immunization for measles, mumps and rubella, *Am. J. Publ. Health*, 75:739–744, 1985.

44. Center for Disease Control, Diphtheria-tetanus-pertussis vaccine shortage — United States, *Mort. Morb. Wk. Rep.*, 33, 695, 1984.

45. Public law 96–660, The National Childhood Vaccine Injury Act of 1986, 1986.

46. World Bank, World Development Report, Oxford University Press (for the World Bank), New York, 1992.

47. Velander W.H., Lubon, H., and Drohan, W., Transgenic livestock as drug factories, *Sci. Am.*, p. 70–74, January 1997.

48. Campbell, K.H.S., McWhir, J., Ritchie, W.A., and Milmut, I., Sheep cloned by nuclear transfer from a cultured cell line, *Nature*, 385:810–813, 1997.

49. Schnieke, E. et al., Human factor IX transgenic sheep produced by transfer of nuclei from transfected fetal fibroblasts, *Science*, 278:2130–2133, 1997.

50. Gibbs, J.B., Mechanism-based target identification and drug discovery in cancer research, *Science*, 287:1969–1973, 2000.

51. Margolis, S. and Carter, H.B. In the *Johns Hopkins White Paper on Prostate Disorders*, Johns Hopkins Medical Institutions, Baltimore, 1997.

52. Garnick, M.B. and Fair, W.R., Prostate cancer, *Sci. Am.*, p. 75–83, December 1998.

53. George-Hyslop, P.H., Piecing together Alzheimer's, *Sci. Am.,* p. 76–83, December 2000.
54. CDC. Update: Investigation of bioterrorism-related anthrax — Connecticut, 2001, *Morb. Mort. Wk. Rep.,* 50:1077–1079, 2001.
55. Inglesby, T.V., Henderson, D.A., Bartlett, J.G. et al., Anthrax as a biological weapon — medical and public health management, *JAMA,* 281:1735–1745, 1999.
56. HHS Fact Sheet. HHS initiative prepares for possible bioterrorism threat. http://www.hhs.gov/news/press/2000pres/20000518.html, May 18, 2000.
57. Cohen, J., and Marshall, E., Vaccines for biodefense: a system in distress, *Science,* 294:498–501, 2001.

APPENDIX

I. GENERAL REGULATIONS FOR DRUGS AND BIOLOGICAL PRODUCTS

Title 21, Code of Federal Regulations (CFR), Chapter I.

A. Part 200–299, Subchapter C — Drugs: General

200 General
210 Current good manufacturing practice in manufacturing, processing, packing, or holding of drugs; general
211 Current good manufacturing practice for finished pharmaceuticals
225 Current good manufacturing practice for medicated feeds
250 Special requirements for specific human drugs
290 Controlled drugs

B. Part 300–499, Subchapter D — Drugs for Human Use

300 General
310 New drugs
312 Investigational new drug application
314 Applications for FDA approval to market a new drug or an antibiotic drug
320 Bioavailability and bioequivalence requirements
330 Over-the-counter (OTC) human drugs, which are generally recognized as safe and effective and not misbranded

C. Part 600–799, Subchapter F — Biologics

600 Biological products: general
601 Licensing
610 General biological product standard
620 Additional standards for bacterial products
630 Additional standards for viral vaccines

D. Others

50   Protection of human subjects
56   Institutional review boards
58   Nonclinical laboratory studies, good laboratory practice (GLP) regulations

The manufacture and distribution of licensed biological products for human use are regulated under the following statutory authorities.

1. Section 351 of the Public Health Service Act (PHS Act)
2. Federal Food, Drug and Cosmetic Act

II. CENTER FOR DRUG EVALUATION AND RESEARCH (CDER), LIST OF IMPORTANT GUIDELINES

For information on a specific guidance document, contact the following office:

Office of Training and Communications,
Division of Drug Information
5600 Fishers Lane
Rockville, MD 20857
Telephone: 301–827–4573
Fax: 301–827–4577
E-mail: druginfo@cder.fda.gov

Guidance (Issue date):

Chemistry

Drug Master Files (I), 9/1/89
Drug Master Files for Bulk Antibiotic Drug Substances (I), 11/29/99
IND Meetings for Human Drugs and Biologics; Chemistry, Manufacturing, and Controls Information (I), 5/25/01
Submitting Documentation for the Manufacturing of and Controls for Drug Products (I), 2/1/87
Analytical Procedures and Methods Validation: Chemistry, Manufacturing, and Controls, 8/30/00
Botanical Drug Products (I), 8/1/00
Stability Testing of Drug Substances and Drug Products (I), 6/8/98

Clinical Medical

Developing Antimicrobial Drugs — General Considerations for Clinical Trials (I), 7/22/98

Acceptance of Foreign Clinical Studies (I), 3/13/01

Compliance

General Principles of Process Validation (I), 5/1/97

Pharmacology/Toxicology

Content and Format of INDs for Phase 1 Studies of Drugs Including Well-Characterized, Therapeutic, Biotechnology-Derived Products (I), 10/4/00

Single-Dose Acute Toxicity Testing for Pharmaceuticals (I), 8/26/96

Immunotoxicity Evaluation of Investigational New Drugs (I), 5/11/01

Retrieve Data   Reset Form

DEPARTMENT OF HEALTH AND HUMAN SERVICES
PUBLIC HEALTH SERVICE
FOOD AND DRUG ADMINISTRATION
INVESTIGATIONAL NEW DRUG APPLICATION (IND)
(TITLE 21, CODE OF FEDERAL REGULATIONS (CFR) PART 312)

Form Approved: OMB No. 0910-0014.
Expiration Date: November 30, 2002
See OMB Statement on Reverse.

NOTE: No drug may be shipped or clinical investigation begun until an IND for that investigation is in effect (21 CFR 312.40).

1. NAME OF SPONSOR

2. DATE OF SUBMISSION

3. ADDRESS *(Number, Street, City, State and Zip Code)*

4. TELEPHONE NUMBER *(Include Area Code)*

5. NAME(S) OF DRUG *(Include all available names: Trade, Generic, Chemical, Code)*

6. IND NUMBER *(If previously assigned)*

7. INDICATION(S) *(Covered by this submission)*

8. PHASE(S) OF CLINICAL INVESTIGATION TO BE CONDUCTED:
☐ PHASE 1 ☐ PHASE 2 ☐ PHASE 3 ☐ OTHER
(Specify)

9. LIST NUMBERS OF ALL INVESTIGATIONAL NEW DRUG APPLICATIONS (21 CFR Part 312), NEW DRUG OR ANTIBIOTIC APPLICATIONS *(21 CFR Part 314)*, DRUG MASTER FILES *(21 CFR Part 314.420)*, AND PRODUCT LICENSE APPLICATIONS (21 CFR Part 601) REFERRED TO IN THIS APPLICATION.

10. *IND submission should be consecutively numbered. The initial IND should be numbered "Serial number: 000." The next submission (e.g., amendment, report, or correspondence) should be numbered "Serial Number: 001." Subsequent submissions should be numbered consecutively in the order in which they are submitted.*

SERIAL NUMBER

11. THIS SUBMISSION CONTAINS THE FOLLOWING: *(Check all that apply)*

☐ INITIAL INVESTIGATIONAL NEW DRUG APPLICATION (IND)   ☐ RESPONSE TO CLINICAL HOLD

PROTOCOL AMENDMENT(S):   INFORMATION AMENDMENT(S):   IND SAFETY REPORT(S):

☐ NEW PROTOCOL   ☐ CHEMISTRY/MICROBIOLOGY   ☐ INITIAL WRITTEN REPORT
☐ CHANGE IN PROTOCOL   ☐ PHARMACOLOGY/TOXICOLOGY   ☐ FOLLOW-UP TO A WRITTEN REPORT
☐ NEW INVESTIGATOR   ☐ CLINICAL

☐ RESPONSE TO FDA REQUEST FOR INFORMATION   ☐ ANNUAL REPORT   ☐ GENERAL CORRESPONDENCE

☐ REQUEST FOR REINSTATEMENT OF IND THAT IS WITHDRAWN,   ☐ OTHER
INACTIVATED, TERMINATED OR DISCONTINUED   *(Specify)*

CHECK ONLY IF APPLICABLE

JUSTIFICATION STATEMENT MUST BE SUBMITTED WITH APPLICATION FOR ANY CHECKED BELOW. REFER TO THE CITED CFR SECTION FOR FURTHER INFORMATION.

☐ TREATMENT IND 21 CFR 312.35(b)   ☐ TREATMENT PROTOCOL 21 CFR 312.35(a)   ☐ CHARGE REQUEST/NOTIFICATION 21 CFR312.7(d)

FOR FDA USE ONLY

CDR/DBIND/DGD RECEIPT STAMP   DDR RECEIPT STAMP   DIVISION ASSIGNMENT:

IND NUMBER ASSIGNED:

FORM FDA 1571 (9/02)   PREVIOUS EDITION IS OBSOLETE.   PAGE 1 OF 2
PSC Media Arts (301) 443-1090   EF

Save Data   Next Page

Figure A.1   Form FDA 1571 (9/02). Investigational New Drug Application (IND)

Previous Page

CONTENTS OF APPLICATION

12.
This application contains the following items: *(Check all that apply)*

☐ 1. Form FDA 1571 *[21 CFR 312.23(a)(1)]*
☐ 2. Table of Contents *[21 CFR 312.23(a)(2)]*
☐ 3. Introductory statement *[21 CFR 312.23(a)(3)]*
☐ 4. General Investigational plan *[21 CFR 312.23(a)(3)]*
☐ 5. Investigator's brochure *[21 CFR 312.23(a)(5)]*
☐ 6. Protocol(s) *[21 CFR 312.23(a)(6)]*
    ☐ a. Study protocol(s) *[21 CFR 312.23(a)(6)]*
    ☐ b. Investigator data *[21 CFR 312.23(a)(6)(iii)(b)]* or completed Form(s) FDA 1572
    ☐ c. Facilities data *[21 CFR 312.23(a)(6)(iii)(b)]* or completed Form(s) FDA 1572
    ☐ d. Institutional Review Board data *[21 CFR 312.23(a)(6)(iii)(b)]* or completed Form(s) FDA 1572
☐ 7. Chemistry, manufacturing, and control data *[21 CFR 312.23(a)(7)]*
    ☐ Environmental assessment or claim for exclusion *[21 CFR 312.23(a)(7)(iv)(e)]*
☐ 8. Pharmacology and toxicology data *[21 CFR 312.23(a)(8)]*
☐ 9. Previous human experience *[21 CFR 312.23(a)(9)]*
☐ 10. Additional information *[21 CFR 312.23(a)(10)]*

13. IS ANY PART OF THE CLINICAL STUDY TO BE CONDUCTED BY A CONTRACT RESEARCH ORGANIZATION? ☐ YES ☐ NO

IF YES, WILL ANY SPONSOR OBLIGATIONS BE TRANSFERRED TO THE CONTRACT RESEARCH ORGANIZATION? ☐ YES ☐ NO

IF YES, ATTACH A STATEMENT CONTAINING THE NAME AND ADDRESS OF THE CONTRACT RESEARCH ORGANIZATION, IDENTIFICATION OF THE CLINICAL STUDY, AND A LISTING OF THE OBLIGATIONS TRANSFERRED.

14. NAME AND TITLE OF THE PERSON RESPONSIBLE FOR MONITORING THE CONDUCT AND PROGRESS OF THE CLINICAL INVESTIGATIONS

15. NAME(S) AND TITLE(S) OF THE PERSON(S) RESPONSIBLE FOR REVIEW AND EVALUATION OF INFORMATION RELEVANT TO THE SAFETY OF THE DRUG

I agree not to begin clinical investigations until 30 days after FDA's receipt of the IND unless I receive earlier notification by FDA that the studies may begin. I also agree not to begin or continue clinical investigations covered by the IND if those studies are placed on clinical hold. I agree that an Institutional Review Board (IRB) that complies with the requirements set fourth in 21 CFR Part 56 will be responsible for initial and continuing review and approval of each of the studies in the proposed clinical investigation. I agree to conduct the investigation in accordance with all other applicable regulatory requirements.

16. NAME OF SPONSOR OR SPONSOR'S AUTHORIZED REPRESENTATIVE

17. SIGNATURE OF SPONSOR OR SPONSOR'S AUTHORIZED REPRESENTATIVE

18. ADDRESS *(Number, Street, City, State and Zip Code)*

19. TELEPHONE NUMBER *(Include Area Code)*

20. DATE

(**WARNING**: A willfully false statement is a criminal offense. U.S.C. Title 18, Sec. 1001.)

Public reporting burden for this collection of information is estimated to average 100 hours per response, including the time for reviewing instructions, searching existing data sources, gathering and maintaining the data needed, and completing reviewing the collection of information. Send comments regarding this burden estimate or any other aspect of this collection of information, including suggestions for reducing this burden to:

Food and Drug Administration	Food and Drug Administration	*An agency may not conduct or sponsor, and a
CBER (HFM-99)	CDER (HFD-94)	person is not required to respond to, a
1401 Rockville Pike	12229 Wilkins Avenue	collection of information unless it displays a
Rockville, MD 20852-1448	Rockville, MD 20852	currently valid OMB control number.*

Please **DO NOT RETURN** this application to this address.

FORM FDA 1571 (9/02)   PAGE 2 OF 2

Save Data   Print   Email Form

Figure A.1 (continued)   Form FDA 1571 (9/02). Investigational New Drug Application (IND)

Retrieve Data   Reset Form

DEPARTMENT OF HEALTH AND HUMAN SERVICES	Form Approved: OMB No. 0910-0014.

DEPARTMENT OF HEALTH AND HUMAN SERVICES
PUBLIC HEALTH SERVICE
FOOD AND DRUG ADMINISTRATION
STATEMENT OF INVESTIGATOR
(TITLE 21, CODE OF FEDERAL REGULATIONS (CFR) PART 312)
(See instructions on reverse side.)

Form Approved: OMB No. 0910-0014.
Expiration Date: November 30, 2002.
See OMB Statement on Reverse.

NOTE: No investigator may participate in an investigation until he/she provides the sponsor with a completed, signed Statement of Investigator, Form FDA 1572 (21 CFR 312.53(c)).

1. NAME AND ADDRESS OF INVESTIGATOR

2. EDUCATION, TRAINING, AND EXPERIENCE THAT QUALIFIES THE INVESTIGATOR AS AN EXPERT IN THE CLINICAL INVESTIGATION OF THE DRUG FOR THE USE UNDER INVESTIGATION. ONE OF THE FOLLOWING IS ATTACHED.

☐ CURRICULUM VITAE   ☐ OTHER STATEMENT OF QUALIFICATIONS

3. NAME AND ADDRESS OF ANY MEDICAL SCHOOL, HOSPITAL OR OTHER RESEARCH FACILITY WHERE THE CLINICAL INVESTIGATION(S) WILL BE CONDUCTED.

4. NAME AND ADDRESS OF ANY CLINICAL LABORATORY FACILITIES TO BE USED IN THE STUDY.

5. NAME AND ADDRESS OF THE INSTITUTIONAL REVIEW BOARD (IRB) THAT IS RESPONSIBLE FOR REVIEW AND APPROVAL OF THE STUDY(IES).

6. NAMES OF THE SUBINVESTIGATORS *(e.g., research fellows, residents, associates)* WHO WILL BE ASSISTING THE INVESTIGATOR IN THE CONDUCT OF THE INVESTIGATION(S).

7. NAME AND CODE NUMBER, IF ANY, OF THE PROTOCOL(S) IN THE IND FOR THE STUDY(IES) TO BE CONDUCTED BY THE INVESTIGATOR.

FORM FDA 1572 (9/02)   PREVIOUS EDITION IS OBSOLETE.   **PAGE 1 OF 2**   PSC Media Arts (301) 443-1090   EF

Save Data   Next Page

Figure A.2   Form FDA 1572 (9/02). Statement of Investigator

Previous Page

8. ATTACH THE FOLLOWING CLINICAL PROTOCOL INFORMATION:

☐ FOR PHASE 1 INVESTIGATIONS, A GENERAL OUTLINE OF THE PLANNED INVESTIGATION INCLUDING THE ESTIMATED DURATION OF THE STUDY AND THE MAXIMUM NUMBER OF SUBJECTS THAT WILL BE INVOLVED.

☐ FOR PHASE 2 OR 3 INVESTIGATIONS, AN OUTLINE OF THE STUDY PROTOCOL INCLUDING AN APPROXIMATION OF THE NUMBER OF SUBJECTS TO BE TREATED WITH THE DRUG AND THE NUMBER TO BE EMPLOYED AS CONTROLS, IF ANY; THE CLINICAL USES TO BE INVESTIGATED; CHARACTERISTICS OF SUBJECTS BY AGE, SEX, AND CONDITION; THE KIND OF CLINICAL OBSERVATIONS AND LABORATORY TESTS TO BE CONDUCTED; THE ESTIMATED DURATION OF THE STUDY; AND COPIES OR A DESCRIPTION OF CASE REPORT FORMS TO BE USED.

9. COMMITMENTS:

I agree to conduct the study(ies) in accordance with the relevant, current protocol(s) and will only make changes in a protocol after notifying the sponsor, except when necessary to protect the safety, rights, or welfare of subjects.

I agree to personally conduct or supervise the described investigation(s).

I agree to inform any patients, or any persons used as controls, that the drugs are being used for investigational purposes and I will ensure that the requirements relating to obtaining informed consent in 21 CFR Part 50 and institutional review board (IRB) review and approval in 21 CFR Part 56 are met.

I agree to report to the sponsor adverse experiences that occur in the course of the investigation(s) in accordance with 21 CFR 312.64.

I have read and understand the information in the investigator's brochure, including the potential risks and side effects of the drug.

I agree to ensure that all associates, colleagues, and employees assisting in the conduct of the study(ies) are informed about their obligations in meeting the above commitments.

I agree to maintain adequate and accurate records in accordance with 21 CFR 312.62 and to make those records available for inspection in accordance with 21 CFR 312.68.

I will ensure that an IRB that complies with the requirements of 21 CFR Part 56 will be responsible for the initial and continuing review and approval of the clinical investigation. I also agree to promptly report to the IRB all changes in the research activity and all unanticipated problems involving risks to human subjects or others. Additionally, I will not make any changes in the research without IRB approval, except where necessary to eliminate apparent immediate hazards to human subjects.

I agree to comply with all other requirements regarding the obligations of clinical investigators and all other pertinent requirements in 21 CFR Part 312.

INSTRUCTIONS FOR COMPLETING FORM FDA 1572
STATEMENT OF INVESTIGATOR:

1. Complete all sections. Attach a separate page if additional space is needed.

2. Attach curriculum vitae or other statement of qualifications as described in Section 2.

3. Attach protocol outline as described in Section 8.

4. Sign and date below.

5. FORWARD THE COMPLETED FORM AND ATTACHMENTS TO THE SPONSOR. The sponsor will incorporate this information along with other technical data into an Investigational New Drug Application (IND).

10. SIGNATURE OF INVESTIGATOR	11. DATE

(WARNING: A willfully false statement is a criminal offense. U.S.C. Title 18, Sec. 1001.)

Public reporting burden for this collection of information is estimated to average 100 hours per response, including the time for reviewing instructions, searching existing data sources, gathering and maintaining the data needed, and completing reviewing the collection of information. Send comments regarding this burden estimate or any other aspect of this collection of information, including suggestions for reducing this burden to:

Food and Drug Administration
CBER (HFM-99)
1401 Rockville Pike
Rockville, MD 20852-1448

Food and Drug Administration
CDER (HFD-94)
12229 Wilkins Avenue
Rockville, MD 20852

"An agency may not conduct or sponsor, and a person is not required to respond to, a collection of information unless it displays a currently valid OMB control number."

Please **DO NOT RETURN** this application to this address.

FORM FDA 1572 (9/02)

PAGE 2 OF 2

Save Data   Print   Email Form

Figure A.2 (continued)   Form FDA 1572 (9/02). Statement of Investigator

DEPARTMENT OF HEALTH AND HUMAN SERVICES FOOD AND DRUG ADMINISTRATION	Form Approved: OMB No. 0910-0338 Expiration Date: August 31, 2005 See OMB Statement on page 2.
APPLICATION TO MARKET A NEW DRUG, BIOLOGIC, **OR AN ANTIBIOTIC DRUG FOR HUMAN USE** (Title 21, Code of Federal Regulations, Parts 314 & 601)	**FOR FDA USE ONLY** APPLICATION NUMBER

APPLICANT INFORMATION

NAME OF APPLICANT	DATE OF SUBMISSION
TELEPHONE NO. (Include Area Code)	FACSIMILE (FAX) Number (Include Area Code)
APPLICANT ADDRESS (Number, Street, City, State, Country, ZIP Code or Mail Code, and U.S. License number if previously issued):	AUTHORIZED U.S. AGENT NAME & ADDRESS (Number, Street, City, State, ZIP Code, telephone & FAX number) IF APPLICABLE

PRODUCT DESCRIPTION

NEW DRUG OR ANTIBIOTIC APPLICATION NUMBER, OR BIOLOGICS LICENSE APPLICATION NUMBER (If previously issued)

ESTABLISHED NAME (e.g., Proper name, USP/USAN name)	PROPRIETARY NAME (trade name) IF ANY
CHEMICAL/BIOCHEMICAL/BLOOD PRODUCT NAME (If any)	CODE NAME (If any)

DOSAGE FORM:	STRENGTHS:	ROUTE OF ADMINISTRATION:

(PROPOSED) INDICATION(S) FOR USE:

APPLICATION INFORMATION

APPLICATION TYPE
(check one) ☐ NEW DRUG APPLICATION (21 CFR 314.50)   ☐ ABBREVIATED NEW DRUG APPLICATION (ANDA, 21 CFR 314.94)
☐ BIOLOGICS LICENSE APPLICATION (21 CFR Part 601)

IF AN NDA, IDENTIFY THE APPROPRIATE TYPE   ☐ 505 (b)(1)   ☐ 505 (b)(2)

IF AN ANDA, OR 505(b)(2), IDENTIFY THE REFERENCE LISTED DRUG PRODUCT THAT IS THE BASIS FOR THE SUBMISSION
Name of Drug   Holder of Approved Application

TYPE OF SUBMISSION (check one)   ☐ ORIGINAL APPLICATION   ☐ AMENDMENT TO A PENDING APPLICATION   ☐ RESUBMISSION
☐ PRESUBMISSION   ☐ ANNUAL REPORT   ☐ ESTABLISHMENT DESCRIPTION SUPPLEMENT   ☐ EFFICACY SUPPLEMENT
☐ LABELING SUPPLEMENT   ☐ CHEMISTRY MANUFACTURING AND CONTROLS SUPPLEMENT   ☐ OTHER

IF A SUBMISSION OF PARTIAL APPLICATION, PROVIDE LETTER DATE OF AGREEMENT TO PARTIAL SUBMISSION: _____

IF A SUPPLEMENT, IDENTIFY THE APPROPRIATE CATEGORY   ☐ CBE   ☐ CBE-30   ☐ Prior Approval (PA)

REASON FOR SUBMISSION

PROPOSED MARKETING STATUS (check one)   ☐ PRESCRIPTION PRODUCT (Rx)   ☐ OVER THE COUNTER PRODUCT (OTC)

NUMBER OF VOLUMES SUBMITTED _____   THIS APPLICATION IS   ☐ PAPER   ☐ PAPER AND ELECTRONIC   ☐ ELECTRONIC

ESTABLISHMENT INFORMATION (Full establishment information should be provided in the body of the Application.)
Provide locations of all manufacturing, packaging and control sites for drug substance and drug product (continuation sheets may be used if necessary). Include name, address, contact, telephone number, registration number (CFN), DMF number, and manufacturing steps and/or type of testing (e.g. Final dosage form, Stability testing) conducted at the site. Please indicate whether the site is ready for inspection or, if not, when it will be ready.

Cross References (list related License Applications, INDs, NDAs, PMAs, 510(k)s, IDEs, BMFs, and DMFs referenced in the current application)

FORM FDA 356h (9/02)
PSC Media Arts (301) 443-1090   EF

PAGE 1

Figure A.3   Form FDA 356h (9/02). Application to Market a New Drug, Biologic, or an Antibiotic Drug for Human Use

	This application contains the following items: *(Check all that apply)*
	1. Index
	2. Labeling *(check one)* ☐ Draft Labeling ☐ Final Printed Labeling
	3. Summary (21 CFR 314.50 (c))
	4. Chemistry section
	A. Chemistry, manufacturing, and controls information (e.g., 21 CFR 314.50(d)(1); 21 CFR 601.2)
	B. Samples (21 CFR 314.50 (e)(1); 21 CFR 601.2 (a)) (Submit only upon FDA's request)
	C. Methods validation package (e.g., 21 CFR 314.50(e)(2)(i); 21 CFR 601.2)
	5. Nonclinical pharmacology and toxicology section (e.g., 21 CFR 314.50(d)(2); 21 CFR 601.2)
	6. Human pharmacokinetics and bioavailability section (e.g., 21 CFR 314.50(d)(3); 21 CFR 601.2)
	7. Clinical Microbiology (e.g., 21 CFR 314.50(d)(4))
	8. Clinical data section (e.g., 21 CFR 314.50(d)(5); 21 CFR 601.2)
	9. Safety update report (e.g., 21 CFR 314.50(d)(5)(vi)(b); 21 CFR 601.2)
	10. Statistical section (e.g., 21 CFR 314.50(d)(6); 21 CFR 601.2)
	11. Case report tabulations (e.g., 21 CFR 314.50(f)(1); 21 CFR 601.2)
	12. Case report forms (e.g., 21 CFR 314.50 (f)(2); 21 CFR 601.2)
	13. Patent information on any patent which claims the drug (21 U.S.C. 355(b) or (c))
	14. A patent certification with respect to any patent which claims the drug (21 U.S.C. 355 (b)(2) or (j)(2)(A))
	15. Establishment description (21 CFR Part 600, if applicable)
	16. Debarment certification (FD&C Act 306 (k)(1))
	17. Field copy certification (21 CFR 314.50 (l)(3))
	18. User Fee Cover Sheet (Form FDA 3397)
	19. Financial Information (21 CFR Part 54)
	20. OTHER *(Specify)*

CERTIFICATION

I agree to update this application with new safety information about the product that may reasonably affect the statement of contraindications, warnings, precautions, or adverse reactions in the draft labeling. I agree to submit safety update reports as provided for by regulation or as requested by FDA. If this application is approved, I agree to comply with all applicable laws and regulations that apply to approved applications, including, but not limited to the following:

1. Good manufacturing practice regulations in 21 CFR Parts 210, 211 or applicable regulations, Parts 606, and/or 820.
2. Biological establishment standards in 21 CFR Part 600.
3. Labeling regulations in 21 CFR Parts 201, 606, 610, 660, and/or 809.
4. In the case of a prescription drug or biological product, prescription drug advertising regulations in 21 CFR Part 202.
5. Regulations on making changes in application in FD&C Act Section 506A, 21 CFR 314.71, 314.72, 314.97, 314.99, and 601.12.
6. Regulations on Reports in 21 CFR 314.80, 314.81, 600.80, and 600.81.
7. Local, state and Federal environmental impact laws.

If this application applies to a drug product that FDA has proposed for scheduling under the Controlled Substances Act, I agree not to market the product until the Drug Enforcement Administration makes a final scheduling decision.

The data and information in this submission have been reviewed and, to the best of my knowledge are certified to be true and accurate.

Warning: A willfully false statement is a criminal offense, U.S. Code, title 18, section 1001.

SIGNATURE OF RESPONSIBLE OFFICIAL OR AGENT	TYPED NAME AND TITLE		DATE
ADDRESS *(Street, City, State, and ZIP Code)*		Telephone Number ( )	

Public reporting burden for this collection of information is estimated to average 24 hours per response, including the time for reviewing instructions, searching existing data sources, gathering and maintaining the data needed, and completing and reviewing the collection of information. Send comments regarding this burden estimate or any other aspect of this collection of information, including suggestions for reducing this burden to:

Department of Health and Human Services Food and Drug Administration CBER, HFM-99 1401 Rockville Pike Rockville, MD 20852-1448	Food and Drug Administration CDER, HFD-94 12420 Parklawn Dr., Room 3046 Rockville, MD 20852	An agency may not conduct or sponsor, and a person is not required to respond to, a collection of information unless it displays a currently valid OMB control number.

FORM FDA 356h (9/02)

PAGE 2

Figure A.3 (continued) Form FDA 356h (9/02). Application to Market a New Drug, Biologic, or an Antibiotic Drug for Human Use

INDEX

A

Absorption, pharmacokinetic models for, 60–62

Acidosis, 131

Adenylate cyclase, activation of, 135

ADME (absorption, distribution, metabolism, and elimination) assessment, 60, 152

Administration route, 12

Adverse drug reaction (ADR), 85–88, 136–137

  causal relationship between drugs and, 137–139

  collection of data in Japan,94–95

  criteria for causality assessment of, 138

  definition of, 85–86

  FDA reports on, 86–88

  monitoring for, 86–88

  during pregnancy and lactation, 139–141

  prevention of, 138–139

  serious, 86

  suffering relief fund law, 96

Advisory committees, 103

Age, drug response and, 131–133

Aging, diseases of, 209–212

Aging population, health goals of, 174–175

Alcohol, 129–130

Allergic reactions, 137

Allopurinol, 2, 134

α2-interferon (alpha), 11

α-tocopherol (alpha), 165

Alternative medicine, 193–194

Alzheimer's disease, 211–212

Aminoglycosides, 134

Aminosalicylic acid, 130

Amobarbital, 149

Analytic reference standard, 68

Analytic techniques, 102

Anesthesia, malignant hyperthermia of, 136

Animal care, 54, 59

Animal safety test, 37

acute toxicity studies, 37

  carcinogenicity study in, 48–50

  mutagenicity study in, 46–48

  reproductive and developmental toxicity studies, 39–46

  subacute and chronic toxicity studies, 38–39

Animal studies, 32

  carcinogenicity, 48–50, 155

  maximum tolerated dose in, 155

Antacids, 128

Antibacterial drugs, 7

Antibiotics

  development of newer generations of, 3

  discovery and development of, 2

  efficacy of, 7–8

Anticholinergics, 4

Anticoagulants, 9, 151

Antihistamines, 150

Antimetabolites, 150

Antimicrobial drugs

  discoveries leading to, 7

  golden age of, 2

Antioxidants, 165

Antipyretics, 130

Antipyrine, 129

Aplastic anemia, chloramphenicol-induced, 136

Approvable letter, 80

Approval letter, 80

Asclepius, 5–6

Ascorbic acid

  as antioxidant, 165

  inactivation of, 133

Ascorbyl palmiate, 165

Asp 79, 135

Autoclaving, 166

B

Baicalain, 188–189

Baicalin, 188–189